"A Homegrown Topeka computer software company that works with national clients is taking a step into the new market: Weight Control for the general public, with a product called "Fat Stats."

-Vickie Griffith Hawver, Healthy Living Editor

FAT STATS

A Guide to Weight Control

Your Personal Trainer and Guide That Provides the Motivation and Information You Need to Take Control of Your Weight Now

David H. Fisher, Jr.

ISBN 0-9644813-0-8

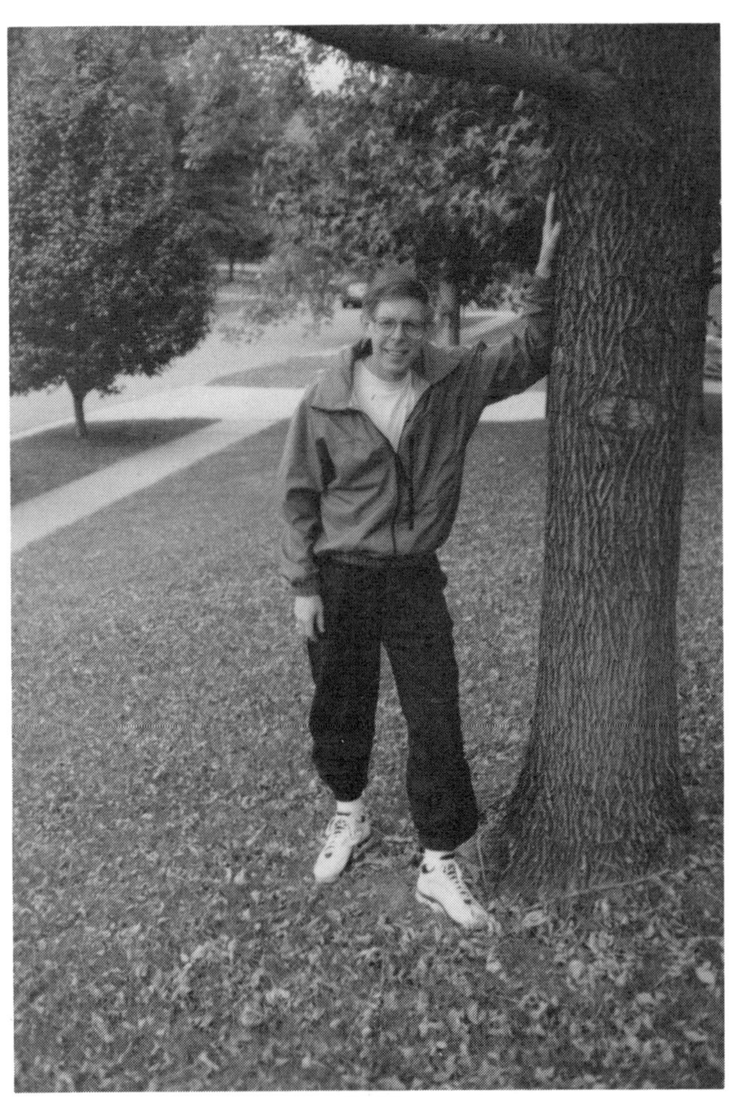

David H. Fisher, Jr., Author

Table of Contents

This book is dedicated to my wife Kathy and our three children: Trey, Shane and Shannan. Without their love, support and advice, this book would not have been possible.

A Dave Fisher, Jr. Productions, Inc. Publication

Dave Fisher, Jr.
Productions, Inc.
3127 SW Huntoon
Topeka, KS 66604

Printed in the United States of America
Second printing December, 1994

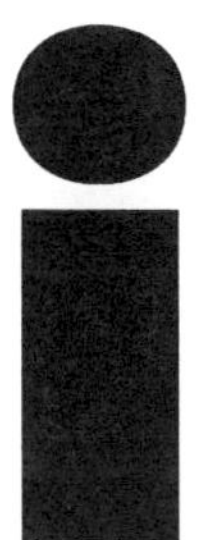

Introduction

My purpose in writing this book is to help people control their weight. I have enjoyed the benefits of maintaining my weight at or near the ideal level all of my adult life. This has not been by accident, I planned it that way! Over the years I have closely monitored my weight on a daily basis. Whenever I have noticed a slight increase I made adjustments in the foods I ate and in my daily activity level. This quickly brought my weight back down.

The material in this book is the result of many years of research as well as my own personal experiences. It will give you insight as to why some people maintain their proper weight while others don't. For example, if you were to ask several overweight people about dieting, each will have his or her own theories, ideas and favorite diets. Since they have not been successful, overweight people are not the ones to consult regarding weight control. It is important to get inside the minds of people who have been successful over the years. They are the ones who hold the keys to successful weight control.

In our modern lifestyle, maintaining an ideal weight doesn't just happen. Many people who control their weight successfully may tell you they don't have a plan, but in almost every case, they do follow certain rules whenever they consume any type of food or beverage.

Don't think of weight control as dieting. Weight control is maintaining good eating habits throughout your lifetime. Weight control should not be an obsession; it is planned eating combined with pursuing your normal daily activities and interests.

To effectively control your weight, you should become familiar with four important factors:

1. *Have a target weight that YOU want to achieve and maintain.*
2. *Understand how to control YOUR weight.*
3. *Make a serious COMMITMENT to accomplish your objective.*
4. *Take immediate ACTION.*

The chapters ahead are designed to help you learn about these factors so you can control your weight throughout your lifetime. The early chapters deal with the psychology of weight control while the latter chapters deal with specific methods of controlling your weight. At the end of the book, you will find "THE NINE KEYS TO WEIGHT CONTROL" and a list of FAT STAT TIPS. These keys and tips can serve as quick reminders. If these are not enough to refresh your memory turn back and reread the appropriate chapters.

Always remember this important fact, people never fail, they produce a result! Up to this point, regardless of the reasons, you have produced a result. You should accept full responsibility for your current weight and rely solely on yourself to change your weight if you desire. However, nothing will happen until you take action. Weight control should not be made complicated. I have purposefully written this book in such a manner so the information will build upon itself. At times, I will repeat bits and pieces of information to reinforce your growing understanding of how you can take control of your weight.

You should read ONLY one chapter per day!!! Read the chapter SLOWLY and PAUSE often to reflect on each idea and how it can apply to you. It's important that you understand and experience the concepts. Start applying the ideas you learn immediately. Please resist the temptation to read more than one chapter per day. By using this technique the principles of weight control will become an important part of your lifestyle.

1 The Problem

Our weight affects our lives in many different ways. You can let your weight control you or you can control your weight. It's your choice. The purpose of this book is to help you take control of your weight. But before we get started, it's important to understand that the only way to control your weight, over the long haul, is to develop good sound eating habits and to continue them throughout your lifetime. Don't be fooled by fad diets, quick weight loss plans or diet pill claims. These are merely crutches that can only lead to short term weight loss. If you don't change your eating habits and outlook on weight control you are almost sure to fail over the long term. Many claims sound good but they are only playing with your emotions; they are not dealing in reality. This is so important, let me state it again. Quick weight loss programs are designed to sound good but they are stating what you want to hear rather than the realities of long term weight control. To be successful you should view weight control as a permanent, life-long process and not just a quick fix.

Almost everyone seems to be interested in controlling his/her weight. In fact, our weight plays an important role in how we feel about ourselves, our self-image, as well as how we feel physically. It plays a part in how we appear to others and dictates what type of clothing we can wear. How much we weigh also affects us financially as our weight can play a major role in the amount we pay for life, health and disability insurance.

Excess body fat is common in our modern day society and contributes to the high cost of health care. Excess body fat can cause certain types of cancer, heart and circulatory disease, joint disease, diabetes, arthritis, high cholesterol, gallstones and chronic depression. In fact, it has been said that if it wasn't for all of the excess body fat in our country we wouldn't be facing a health care crisis today!

Recent estimates indicate that approximately 34 million adults are 20 percent above their desired weight and are considered overweight. With the emphasis on fast food and computer games, we have also seen a major increase in the body fat levels of our children. It's interesting to note that the earlier the onset of obesity, the greater the likelihood of remaining obese throughout life. This has become a creeping problem that in a few years could be a very serious one for the overall health of our society.

Being overweight places an extra burden on just about every body system. As a person gains more and more weight, fat begins to accumulate around the chest area. When this occurs lung and diaphragm movement is impaired, and it becomes increasingly difficult to breathe. This puts extra strain on the heart and aggravates or worsens respiratory problems such as influenza, pneumonia and obstructive lung disease which are all illnesses that can ultimately lead to death.

Extra fat around the abdomen can put increased pressure on the stomach forcing its contents back into the esophagus, causing heartburn. If you eat a meal that contains alot of fat, you can be left feeling bloated and uncomfortable, since fat takes longer to leave the stomach than protein and carbohydrates. Low-fat foods are easier on the stomach and therefore improve the digestion process.

Few of today's occupations require vigorous physical activity, and much of our leisure time is spent in sedentary activity. This combined with our hectic way of life and the availability of fast food restaurants makes it difficult for us to control our weight.

It should be pointed out that some athletes and many weight trainers are quite muscular and weigh more than the average person for their age and height.

However, their body composition, the amount of fat versus lean body mass (lean body mass consisting of muscle, bone, organs and tissue) is within a desirable range. Others weigh less than the average person but carry around too much fat. The addition of exercise to a weight control program can help control both body weight and body fat.

Of course a certain amount of body fat is necessary for everyone. The normal percentage of fat for women should be around 19%; 16% for men. Women with more than 30% fat and men with more than 20% fat are considered obese.

Weight control should always be kept in the right perspective. Since weight control is only possible by developing and maintaining correct eating habits, it's important to keep in mind that you should always eat a well balanced, nutritional diet. You should guard against any type of eating disorder. Many people have become so obsessed with their weight that they have developed eating disorders such as anorexia (self-induced starvation) and bulimia (binge eating followed by self-induced vomiting). This type of inappropriate eating behavior is not necessary to control your weight and should not be used. It is important to maintain your proper percentage of body fat. You don't want it to be too low any more than you want it to be too high.

Why do you want to control your weight? Do you want to look better both to yourself and to others? Do you want to feel better? Has your doctor advised you to lose weight to help lower blood pressure or for other health reasons? Do you want to get back into the clothes you used to wear a few years ago? Do you want to do everything you can to prevent stroke or diseases such as cancer, heart disease and diabetes? All of these are sound reasons why you should develop a lifetime weight control program.

2 Why People Fail

It was a beautiful day in Kansas. The feeling of spring was in the air. The people I had met were among the happiest I had ever observed. They all had smiles on their faces, and it was obvious that they enjoyed their work. Everyone appeared to be at or near their ideal weight and walked with what I would call perfect posture.

The three and one-half hours of training had been extremely thorough. The G-Suit fit perfectly. The forty pounds of equipment I was carrying on my back was hardly noticed during the two and a half block walk. My adrenaline was pumping so hard that the two story climb up the ladder was easy. The straps and belts were so tight I could hardly move. Then the electronics came to life. The oxygen started to flow and the Pratt & Whitney J-75 Turbojet began to whine. Soon the REPUBLIC F-105 Thunderchief jet fighter taxied to the take-off position. The canopies were closed tight and we were receiving 100 percent pure oxygen.

Major Tart gave full power, lit the afterburner, and 26,500 pounds of thrust slammed us back into our seats as we bolted off into the wild blue yonder. Soon the power was reduced and we climbed to 32,000 feet. Our speed indicator read .70 MACH - (MACH 1.0 is the speed of sound). Upon receiving clearance, Major Tart lit the afterburner again. Even in level flight, the acceleration was incredible. The speed indicator read-out began to increase - .80 MACH - .90 MACH. At this point our acceleration became more difficult. It felt as if we were going through mud or snow in a car - .95 MACH - .97 MACH - .98 MACH - .99 MACH. Next, the readouts on the altimeter and speed indicator began to shake and we burst through the sound barrier. Once again we felt a sensation of tremendous acceleration. At Mach 1.10 Major Tart cut back the power and we flew smoothly and quietly above the speed of sound. For him it was almost routine, for me it was the experience of a lifetime - a dream come true. After an aerial "Dog Fight" with another F-105, low altitude runs, and experiencing G-Forces reaching 4.8 times the weight of gravity, we returned to McConnell Air Force Base in Wichita.

During my two hour drive back to Topeka I thought about the many exciting experiences of the day. I was very impressed by the outstanding quality of the Kansas Air National Guard personnel, the excellent pre-flight training I had been given, and the important role the National Guard plays in the security and freedom of the United States. Suddenly it occurred to me that the process of breaking the sound barrier is like the process of going through the barriers we encounter in life. As we get closer to our goal, the going gets tougher and tougher. However, when we finally break through, like breaking the sound barrier, there is a sense of calm and joy and life takes on new meanings.

You may have tried different types of diets in the past only to have success elude you when the going got tough. The process of changing your eating habits and the way you think about food requires planning combined with action. As you monitor your weight you will experience ups and downs. During the early stages losing weight can be fairly easy, but as you get closer and closer to your goal the temptations you experience will make your goal tougher and tougher to achieve. Yet, like going through the sound barrier, when you finally reach your ideal weight, life can take on new meanings full of fresh experiences, accomplishments, excitement and wonder. When the going gets tough just think how you will feel when you finally attain your ideal weight. You will feel better about your accomplishment than you can imagine!

Now let's get started on the road to controlling your weight. Remember that weight control isn't just a goal, it's a way of life! People fail to control their weight for basically one reason, they take in more calories than they burn, and they do it on a regular basis. This is not a revolutionary idea, it's just a fact. Not long ago I saw a ladies sweatshirt with, "I'M CONSCIOUS OF CALORIES - I EAT THEM AS LONG AS I'M CONSCIOUS!" printed on it. There are a lot of jokes about losing weight and dieting. However, weight control is very serious to those who want to achieve and maintain their ideal weight.

The only way to control our weight is to learn how to balance the calories we eat (energy intake) with the calories we burn (energy output). The underlying causes of obesity and its treatments are complex, but the concept of energy balance is quite simple. If we eat more calories than our body needs to perform our day's activities, the extra calories are stored as fat. On the other hand, if we do not take in enough calories to meet our body's energy needs, our body will go to its stored fat to make up the difference. There are many reasons why people eat too much. Some of the most common reasons are:

1. *They sit down to a good meal and eat too fast. Then, because they enjoyed it so much, they get a second helping and continue eating until they are "STUFFED".*
2. *They are in the habit of cleaning their plate even when they are full.*
3. *They feel obligated to eat more than they want while eating dinner at a friend's home.*
4. *They eat dessert though they are no longer*

hungry just because it is offered to them.

5. *They allow themselves to be influenced by others. How many times have you been told, "Oh, have a piece of my cake!"*
6. *They don't say "no" when offered food because they don't want to hurt someone's feelings.*
7. *They skip a meal to lose weight and become so hungry that they overeat. Often they eat fast and don't feel full until it's TOO LATE!*
8. *They overeat on holidays, birthdays and special occasions.*
9. *They eat when they are stressed or bored.*
10. *They don't weigh themselves every day and therefore they are not aware that they are gaining weight.*
11. *They are on vacation or at a convention and tend to eat and drink more than usual. This is usually combined with doing less than their normal exercise.*
12. *After a hard week's work, they celebrate the arrival of the weekend by overeating.*
13. *They eat the wrong kinds of food.*
14. *When they allow themselves to get extremely hungry, they often desire the wrong kinds of food.*
15. *They have no eating plan, so they eat whenever food is available.*
16. *They don't know what their ideal weight is, so they have no goal or target weight.*
17. *They don't know how many calories they burn so they have no guide to follow.*
18. *They have that proverbial first chip and then can't stop eating them. This is called the "You*

can't just eat one chip" Syndrome.

19. *They drink too much alcohol and don't care what type of food or how much of it they eat.*
20. *They allow their blood sugar to get too low and then eat too much too fast.*

The reasons people consume too much food are not new, and we have all experienced overeating from time to time. Those people who consistently overeat do so because they don't have a weight control or eating plan they can understand. With a good weight control plan and the proper attitude, all of these incorrect eating situations can easily be overcome.

However, in developing a weight control plan it's important to realize that people naturally tend to gain weight as they get older. The cause of this is the fact that their bodies use fewer calories to sustain life, and because they are probably less physically active. Therefore, they burn fewer calories, and if they don't reduce their calorie intake accordingly, they will gain weight. It's very important to know how many calories you burn as you get older so you will know how many calories you should eat.

As you read this book, you will discover how to overcome eating problems and control your weight throughout your lifetime. Let's start by looking at a very important factor, COMMITMENT.

3 Commitment

People who have not succeeded in controlling their weight HAVE NOT MADE A COMMITMENT to follow a weight control plan! WITHOUT A PERSONAL COMMITMENT WE ARE ALMOST SURE TO FAIL. I'm not talking about a casual commitment. I'm talking about a definite commitment to control your weight. I can not stress this enough. YOU MUST MAKE A FIRM COMMITMENT TO CONTROL YOUR WEIGHT. The world is full of heavy people who have tried to reach and maintain their ideal weight but failed because they did not make a commitment. There are some people who feel they need to make their commitment to someone else by reporting to them each week. This should not be necessary. You should make your commitment to yourself and not to someone else. People who control their weight successfully don't rely on anyone else, they take control themselves.

Choose the dream and, from that point on, the dream will change your life. But you can't enjoy the satisfaction of accomplishment until you get started. Oliver Wendell Holmes once said, "I find the great thing in this world is not so much where we stand, as in what direction we are moving." Success is not a destination, it's a journey. Before beginning a new and exciting adventure into controlling your weight, you should prepare yourself. It's hard to notice that you have formed bad habits until you try to break them. Most people get discouraged before they ever reach any type of goal so it's important to re-think your eating habits and to maintain an open mind. To illustrate what I mean, let's consider the following story that I was told a few years ago.

A teacher once invited one of her students over to her house. After a nice visit, the teacher offered the student a diet cola which he accepted. The teacher poured the cola into the student's glass. Even after the glass was full, the teacher continued to pour. Soon the glass overflowed and cola spilled out onto the table. Finally, the student said, "You must stop pouring! The cola is overflowing, it's not going into my glass!" The teacher replied, "You are very observant, and the same is true with you. If you are going to benefit from my teaching, you must first empty out what you have in your mental glass."

As you prepare to study the information in this book, you should keep this same concept in mind. In order to change your thinking about weight control, you must first empty out what you already have in your mental glass: your preconceived ideas. Without the ability to temporarily forget what we know, our minds remain cluttered with old ideas and habit patterns. If we don't keep an open mind, we will never have an opportunity to ask the questions that lead to new ideas.

If you have not been successful in controlling your weight, be prepared and willing to look at the subject differently. The information you uncover in this book should be applied to your personal eating habits in your own creative way without being limited by your old ideas. You may need to break out of the concept prisons you have built regarding how you consume food. You may need to look at food, in general, in a different way and liberate yourself from your old ways of dealing with your desire for food. Begin stimulating new ways to enjoy what you eat. See yourself as an explorer or detective discovering new techniques in reshaping your eating habits. Remember, people are never trapped into continuing to do things as before. Understanding this fact can lead to changes in your attitude and approach to the whole concept of weight control and life.

As you consider the way you have looked at controlling your weight in the past, it's important to realize that there really are definite ways to control your weight. Other people have done it successfully and so can you. In fact, there are many plans you can develop to control your weight. You will find many ideas in this book, and you may be stimulated to invent some new ones on your own. One of the most exciting realities of life is that as you let go of old habits and ideas you are free to look for new ones.

When you discover some ideas about controlling your weight ask yourself the question, "What if I did that?" This is an easy way to get your imagination going and may lead to ways you can apply the information to your own weight control program. For example, what if you didn't eat that piece of cake or waited 30 seconds between bites? What-ifs are ways to free yourself from deeply ingrained assumptions in your eating habits. It allows you to think in different ways. Remember you not only want to generate new ways of controlling your weight, but you also want to escape your old methods.

You may want to look forwards or backwards to see the effect of your eating patterns. For example, when considering eating a piece of pie, you may want to look forward into the future and ask, "How will I feel 30 minutes from now if I eat this piece of pie? Or you may want to look backwards after overeating to discover why you over ate. What did you think about or do that lead to your over consumption of food? Be you own detective and learn from your discoveries.

Don't feel guilty or get discouraged with little setbacks along the road to developing new eating habits. Don't create a catastrophe out of a single mistake. Instead, develop the habit of learning from your failures while benefiting from your successes. Feel good about both your successes and your failures. You are learning each step of the way as you gain control of your weight. If you get discouraged, you probably want the end result too soon. Allow yourself time to learn from your experiences. Keep trying; those who eventually succeed keep at it until they develop a plan that works for them.

Remember, each of the current attitudes you now possess regarding your own weight were developed, programmed, adjusted, and reinforced by you alone. Your attitudes are the result of your own self-talk. No one else can develop your attitude, only you can. Therefore, you must be willing to put aside your current ideas and attitudes so that you are free to consider new ones.

Right now you tend to behave in a manner that is consistent with your self-image. You tend to act like you have in the past over and over again. The point is, you don't tend to act on the basis of your potential but on how you perceive yourself. Don't think, "I wish I could control my weight." We tend to use the word wish for things that we don't feel we can do. There is no question that you can control your weight. This is not wishful thinking. However, you must make the decision that you will take control. Develop a plan and stick with it.

When you decide to control your weight and start following your plan, the success process will begin at once. However, some of your old patterns of behavior will still be there for some time. Remind yourself that you are moving toward your goal and how you will feel when you reach your ideal weight. Lasting change in human behavior is the result of a changed self-image. This change process is not an instantaneous event. You MUST keep working on it!

The most important thing to do, prior to changing your eating habits, is to make the personal commitment that YOU ARE GOING TO CONTROL YOUR WEIGHT and that you will do it consistently. You should keep this in mind and see yourself succeeding. Without a personal commiment all the information you can learn about weight control will probably not successfully help you over the long haul. You will be reminded of this significant truth time and time again as you read this book. Please don't overlook this vital fact!

Recently I talked to a woman about weight control and she informed me that she is so uncomfortable with her weight she closes her eyes whenever she gets out of the shower so she won't have to see herself in the mirror. It's too bad people allow themselves to think like this. How much we weigh is one part of our lives we can control; yet the majority of men and women never take advantage of this important fact.

For most people, maintaining their ideal weight doesn't just happen, they must plan to control their weight and follow their plan on a daily basis. Almost everyone tries to lose weight at some point each year. Even people who do not have a weight problem gain weight from time to time and decide that they need to shed some pounds. Some people are successful with their weight reduction and keep the weight off, while others either never lose much weight or gain it right back and give up. The important fact to remember is that if you don't eat a controlled diet and monitor your weight, chances are you will not maintain your ideal weight. You can't eat whatever you want, whenever you want! But, you can eat and enjoy most of your favorite foods.

Unless you have a health problem, it is very important that you eat some of your favorite foods. However to consume these foods you must put them into your overall plan. For example, my wife and I enjoy eating Mexican food. There is a little family owned restaurant in Topeka called Rosa's. The restaurant is so popular that it's very difficult to get in during normal meal times without a long wait. People come from all over the area to enjoy their delicious food. It is purely a family restaurant with only twelve tables, and they do not serve any type of alcoholic beverage. There is no waiting area inside Rosa's. People line up outside, in all kinds of weather, waiting for the next available table. As soon as you finish your meal, you feel obligated to leave quickly so that the next customers can come in and be seated.

Almost every Saturday morning my wife and I

arrive at Rosa's about 11:00 A.M. so that we'll be sure to get a table. Usually by the time we finish eating lunch, all the tables are full. The reason I mention this is that I can enjoy the food at Rosa's because I plan for this meal. I am very careful to monitor my calories and grams of fat so that I will not exceed my allotment for the day. I allow myself to enjoy this type of food only once a week. You too can control your weight and enjoy your favorite foods by including them in your overall plan.

Why do people gain weight? Again, because they eat too much, that is they consume more calories than they burn. Why they eat too much is another matter. Numerous books have been written on the subject of dieting. Many are technical and the reader often gets discouraged with all of the complicated and confusing information. This book takes the opposite approach. It provides practical information for people who want to control their weight and get results. It's for people who want to begin eating right immediately.

Several years ago I met a man who worked at the local YMCA. He was obviously overweight. I visited with him on several occasions each week during my workouts. One day the subject of fried foods came up. He indicated to me that he loved all types of fried food and ate them on a regular basis. He then made a comment I will never forget. He said, "Some people eat to live, I live to eat." He said he didn't care how much he weighed. He obviously was committed to food rather than physical health and weight control. To accomplish our ideal weight, it is important that you make the commitment to control your eating habits.

When my oldest son, Trey, was in the sixth grade he asked me to coach his Optimist/YMCA basketball team. Though I got my degree in physical education, I didn't know much about coaching basketball. I decided if I was going to do a good job coaching the team I needed to learn from one of the best basketball coaches in the area. I contacted a very successful high school basketball coach for advice and he graciously agreed to meet with me over coffee.

During our meeting I explained everything I could about the individual players I would be coaching and asked for his input. He outlined all of the fundamental skills I should teach the boys and described the best drill to develop each skill. He then outlined the offense and defense I should use and how each position should be played.

I took this information home and studied it carefully. I then taught the players each skill followed by the offensive and defensive strategies, exactly as the high school coach instructed. The end result was that the team won every game by a large margin. The biggest victory was 54 to 0.

I sought out someone who was very successful and learned from him. I then applied this information to my own situation. This is the same point I want to make about weight control. Don't seek advice from people who have been unsuccessful in controlling their weight. Learn from people who have been successful.

The motivation to reach your ideal weight should be to look better, feel better, and improve your health and quality of life. Your main reason for losing weight should not be to look good at your upcoming high school reunion. Your plans will probably backfire because you don't have a meaningful and permanent reason to lose weight and keep it off. Your goal should not be to lose the weight too rapidly, but to develop new eating patterns you can enjoy. Before beginning any weight control or exercise program, it's important to consult your physician.

Now that you are aware of the importance of commitment, you may want to look back at your previous attempts and or successes at controlling your weight to uncover where you failed or why you succeeded.

4 Your Character

As I have already stated, to be successful at weight control you must have a plan, and you must make a commitment to follow it. Let me restate this in a different way. The most important part of weight control takes place from the neck up. You must mentally decide that you are going to take control of your weight.

Remember this: what you do today will determine your weight tomorrow! Another very powerful fact you should keep in mind is WHAT YOU DO TODAY WILL DETERMINE YOUR CHARACTER TOMORROW! If you carefully monitor your weight today and consume the correct amount of calories and fat, then tomorrow you will have the character of a person who carefully monitors his or her weight and eats properly. It will therefore be natural to continue monitoring your weight and eating the correct amount of calories and fat, because it has become a part of your character. However, if you don't monitor your weight today and you eat too many calories and grams of fat, then tomorrow you will have the character of a person who does not eat correctly. Therefore it will seem natural not to monitor your weight, calories and fat.

Because this is so very important let me give you a powerful example. Think back to your school days when a teacher would announce on Monday that you would be given a test the following Friday. You made the decision you wanted to get an "A" on the exam. So, you decided to study two hours every night from 7:00 P.M. to 9:00 P.M., Monday through Thursday. By Friday, with a total of eight hours study time, you felt certain that you would get an "A" on the exam. If you followed your plan and studied for those two hours on Monday evening, you felt good about studying during those same hours every other evening; therefore, it became natural for you to continue this study schedule each evening resulting in that "A" you desired.

On the other hand, if when Monday evening arrived you went out for a pizza and didn't get home until late, you probably decided that it was too late. You shrugged off this failure to follow through with your plan thinking you could make up Monday's time by studying an additional two hours on Tuesday evening. Yet, when Tuesday night arrived you failed to follow your study plan again because of a developing pattern of procrastination. At this point, you ACTUALLY NEEDED A CHANGE IN CHARACTER JUST TO DO YOUR HOMEWORK! Otherwise, you may have put off your studies until Thursday evening. Finally, when the last night to study had arrived, you had to either cram for the exam, or else you decided that there wasn't enough time to study for it resulting in a grade that was far below your expectations.

When the time came for another exam you probably repeated this disastrous pattern, because once you do something you tend to repeat it. What you do today will determine your character tomorrow.

Learning to control your weight requires the same kind of discipline as maintaining the successful study schedule described above. You should develop a plan and stick with it. If you do, it will be easier to develop the personal qualities that will allow you to stick with a weight control plan. However, if you stop and start a diet plan without reaching your goal, you may never be successful in keeping your weight under control. You have probably heard of "YO-YO" diets, where people lose weight for a while and then go back to old eating habits that cause them to gain their weight back. Surprising as it may be, "YO-YO" diets are more detrimental to your body than just staying overweight. Reports indicate that after five years ten percent of those people who have lost substantial amounts of weight have gained the weight back! You need to develop the kind of character that is willing to monitor your weight, calories, and fat grams on a daily basis; even after you have attained your ideal weight. Think of yourself as a person who is in control of his weight, and accept nothing less.

There will be times when you eat too much, though they should be few and far between if you are committed to controlling your weight. When you eat too much and you're monitoring your weight, you can quickly make adjustments and get back on track. You should assume total responsibility if you overeat. Don't give up! Ask yourself: "What lead me to overeat? Was I tired or bored? Did I allow myself to get too hungry? How can I handle it the next time?" Evaluate the situation, and take responsibility by trying to prevent another overeating occurrence.

You should weigh yourself each day so that you can IMMEDIATELY observe the slightest changes in your weight. When your weight is up slightly, make the necessary adjustments quickly.

When you start your plan, keep a diary of your weight and what you eat. Record everything you eat and why you ate it. For example, did you eat this food because you were hungry, because someone offered it to you, or did you eat it because you were nervous? From time to time, review your diary to determine when, what, and why you ate. Soon you will discover your weaknesses, and you will be able to use this knowledge in developing a plan to overcome them.

Remember, the most important aspect of weight control is making a commitment to a plan followed by developing the type of character that will help you live up to your commitment. You can not expect others to be of much help. Misery loves company. People who are overweight will not worry about your weight, while people who control their weight, will seldom suggest another cookie or a piece of cake. After all, they will be eating according to their plan. They would advise you to do the same. They know the effort they put into controlling their weight is far less than the pain of being overweight. Controlling their weight is a part of their character.

5 Visualization

It's very important to visualize how you will look when you reach your ideal weight. Review in your mind, how you are going to deal with problem eating situations, and see yourself handling them in a way that enables you to stick to your plan.

Let me give you a personal example of how the visualization process can work. For eleven years I served as the volunteer swimming coach at the Topeka YMCA. I coached both boys and girls ages six to seventeen. There were five age groups: 8 & Under, 9 & 10, 11 & 12, 13 & 14 and 15-17. We developed many outstanding swimmers and took them to the National YMCA Swimming and Diving Championships almost every year. I started my first year with 16 boys and by the time I quit, the team had grown to over 115 boys and girls. Our swimming season was very long, lasting from October to April, or about the entire school year. We participated in swimming meets approximately twice a month. Each swimmer participated in three individual events and the fastest four boys and four girls in each of the age divisions swam on the 2 relay teams.

Each time a swimmer improved in all three of his or her individual events in one meet, they were given a white star to sew on their team swim suit. If the swimmer was also on a relay team, the relay team had to record their best time for the season, or the relay members didn't receive a white star even if they improved their other times.

Each swimmer practiced about one hour, three times a week. I kept very accurate records on each swimmer's best times and these were updated on a big record board on the wall of the YMCA after each meet. From these records I would select the swimmers who would swim in the relays for their respective age groups.

One week prior to a meet, in the middle of the season, I decided to introduce the visualization process to the team. It's important to remember that the swimmers had trained for several months and were all in excellent condition. Therefore it was difficult for them to improve their times on a regular basis. I wanted to use the visualization process to see how many of the team members could improve their times in all of their events. Remember, I was dealing with boys and girls as young as six and as old as seventeen.

We had a total of 115 boys and girls on the team and each would swim in three individual events for a total of 345 swimming events. In addition, there were two relays in each of the five age groups for an additional ten events. Therefore there would be a maximum of 355 times that could be improved during the meet. Each swimmer selected the three events they were going to swim, and I informed them who would be swimming in the relays. Swimming practice lasted for three hours with each group practicing for about one hour.

As the groups arrived for practice I had them sit down, close their eyes, and we began the visualization process. They started by visualizing themselves arriving at the pool on the day of the meet feeling stronger than they had ever felt before. As their event was called they reported to the starter feeling confident that they would improve their times by swimming the best race of their lives. As they shot off the blocks they reached out further than they had ever reached before hitting the water with tremendous power.

They visualized the feeling of incredible speed as they sliced through the water. When they hit the end of the pool and executed their turns, they could feel their bodies cutting through the water with the mighty force of their push off. I had them swimming the races in their minds, feeling the exhilaration as they swam their final laps. Upon completing the race, each swimmer looked up at the timer, and with the crowd roaring its approval, all of them received the news that they had improved their personal best time. They then visualized climbing out of the pool, experiencing the awesome feeling of accomplishment. The crowd continued to cheer as the swimmer's new record time was announced over the public address system.

We continued this process of visualization for each event concluding with experiencing the wonderful feeling of accomplishment as they are handed the white star for improvement in all their events. This whole process took around ten minutes. We then conducted practice with each swimmer practicing these same feelings while swimming their training laps. I repeated this visualization training for a total of three practices.

On the Saturday of the meet just prior to the swimming events, I met with the entire team consisting of all 115 swimmers. We went through the visualization process one more time together, and each swimmer was asked to repeat the process, alone, prior to swimming their events.

When the meet was over, I was amazed to discover that every swimmer on the team had improved all of their times, including all ten relay teams. Each swimmer had earned a white star. I'll never forget the looks on the faces of the swimmers' parents as I conducted the white star awards ceremony and presented a white star to every swimmer.

There was another interesting thing that I noticed

about this visualization experience. This meet took place in the middle of the winter, during the height of the cold and flu season when we would normally expect five to ten percent of the swimmers to be out sick. However, not one of the 115 swimmers was sick during the one and one half weeks of the visualization training. It's amazing what the power of positive thinking can do!

I tell you this story because I want to stress the importance of positive visualization as you progress through your weight control program. How you visualize controlling your weight is very important. Your self-talk can make the difference in your success or failure. You should always look at the positive side. If you need to lose twenty five pounds and you lose one pound, see yourself as having already lost one pound rather than having twenty four pounds to lose. This will provide positive inspiration, and one little spark of inspiration is at the heart of all accomplishment. At the beginning of every success is the decision to do it followed by visualizing yourself accomplishing your goal. So keep an open mind. Visualize yourself as a person who is controlling his weight. Practice seeing yourself handling all the temptations as they arise, and experience feeling good when you accomplish each goal.

6 Overeating

The major reason people gain weight is that they overeat. Some people would say they overeat because they don't have any will power. Will power is the straining to deny yourself and usually feels like punishment. People eat too much, not because they don't have any will power, but because they don't have a plan to keep from overeating, whether it is subconscious or intentional.

All overeating situations are basically the same. To discover how to keep from overeating, let's look at perhaps the biggest challenge people face, THE THANKSGIVING MEAL. For people who have a weight problem, this is one time they feel it is OK to eat as much as they want. Then they complain because they feel uncomfortable and depressed. For people who control their weight, Thanksgiving is one of their biggest challenges. Everyone wants to enjoy the Thanksgiving meal, but enjoying it does not mean you have to overeat. One helpful way to keep from overeating is to get in back of the line if the meal is being served buffet style. On the other hand, if the food is being passed around the table, be polite and pass the food to the person next to you, asking them to help themselves first. Have them continue to pass the food around the table so you will be last. Someone always has to be first and someone must be last. You should try to be last.

By the time you fill your plate, the others who were served before you will be well into their meal. When you put your food on your plate, be sure not to exceed the amount of food you plan to eat. Then eat your food SLOWLY and enjoy it. By the time you finish your food, the others should have already finished. Make a decision you will not have a second helping until at least 20 minutes after finishing the food on your plate. Your brain needs 20 minutes to register that you are full. By that time the others will have finished their second helping. Most important of all, you will probably no longer be hungry. The feeling of fullness will have arrived in your brain.

Dessert is usually a part of most Thanksgiving meals which adds many unwanted extra calories. If you feel like having dessert, wait 20 minutes before indulging. If you still can't resist the desserts, just have a small amount, eat it very slowly and don't go back for seconds.

When eating any meal it's extremely important to eat your food slowly. Chew your food thoroughly and take time between bites. If you can't control the speed you eat, make sure half the foods you put on your plate are low in calories such as: raw celery, carrots, cauliflower and broccoli. These foods take a longer time to chew, so eat these foods first. They will tend to fill you up and you won't eat as much.

Chew each mouthful slowly and put your fork down between bites. Concentrate on enjoying the flavor of the food rather than just stuffing it down. You will enjoy the eating experience more, and you will feel full and satisfied on less food. At some point in your meal, pause for 30 seconds before going on. Actually time yourself. Then try longer periods. Just think, if you eat your food at half speed, you can enjoy one plate of food over the same period you would normally consume two. When you are tempted to give in, recall the times you have successfully resisted temptation. This will help you resist again. These same ideas will work in any eating situation. The important thing you need to do is, make the decision you will control the amount of food you eat and develop a plan for the meal. Follow your plan!

Another problem we face when going to a party or gathering is what to do about the snacks and hors d'oeuvres. There are several things you can do to keep from eating fattening snacks. Obviously, the most important thing is to make the commitment that you will not eat the snacks. After you make the commitment, there are several things that will help you stick to your plan.

Prior to going to a party where you may be tempted to eat too much, you can help curb your appetite by drinking water and eating raw vegetables. Again, the foods you should consider are: carrots, broccoli, celery or cauliflower. You could substitute the vegetables with fruit. This will fill your stomach with very low calorie snacks so you won't be as tempted to eat fattening foods. Don't drink fruit juices, instead eat fresh fruit. There is nothing wrong with fruit juice, but it takes longer to eat a piece of fresh fruit. You will obtain the satisfaction of chewing while adding fiber to your diet. Of course, if these types of snacks are available at the party, by all means partake of them while you are there.

While at the party, a good rule of thumb is to stay at least an arms length away from the refreshment table so you won't be tempted to eat as much. Preferably keep the refreshments out of sight. Focus your attention on the people who are at the party rather than the food. Many times people eat at parties because they are nervous or bored. If you need something to do at the party, eat a few vegetables or drink a diet beverage. If you take food you don't like, don't finish the plate. Chewing gum is also an option. You can't chew gum and eat at the same time.

If you are going to have your meal at the party, try to eat the same types of food you would eat at home.

Rather than build a big turkey sandwich, have slices of turkey. Put the amount of food you should eat on your plate the first time. Take your time eating and don't go back for seconds. If you are tempted to go back, make the decision that you won't go back for at least 20 minutes. By that time, you probably won't feel like eating anyway.

Remember, be kind to the others, don't bring fattening foods to the party. Take something low calorie and healthy, such as dip based on non-fat yogurt, cottage cheese or ricotta. That way you will not be tempted to eat some fattening food while preparing it.

Keep in mind that alcohol is full of "empty" or "invisible" calories. In addition, alcohol will stimulate your appetite and may lower your ability to resist fattening foods. Have a seltzer with a twist of lemon or lime. No one will know what you are drinking and you will save around 70 to 150 calories. If you must have alcohol, have a low calorie glass of wine or wine spritzer. Alternate them with sparkling water or diet soda. Keep the thought in your mind how happy you will be when you leave the party knowing that you stuck to your plan. Others may leave wishing they hadn't eaten or drunk so much, while you continued to control your weight.

When you get down to your ideal weight, people will be commending you on how good you look and asking how you've controlled your weight. This should give you even more motivation to continue your weight control program. Everyone will expect you to continue maintaining your ideal weight including yourself.

Remember, to keep from overeating, stay away from fattening salad dressings. You have probably seen people going through a buffet line filling up on low calorie salad, only to put fattening dressing on top. Dressing and dip for vegetables probably defeat more diets than any other single food. Two tablespoons of regular high-fat salad dressing contains nearly as much fat as a hamburger. Try putting some fresh fruit on top of your salad or lemon with herbs and spices instead of dressing.

If you must use dressing, try putting a low calorie dressing in a spray bottle and lightly spray it over your salad. This will spread the dressing evenly over your salad without using very much. When eating out or at home have your dressing served on the side and dip your fork into it before spearing the lettuce or vegetables. You'll still get the taste without eating as much dressing. Note the amount of dressing left over after you have finished your salad. The more you have left the more fat and calories you saved.

Margarine has around the same number of calories as butter (about 100 calories per tablespoon). It's easy to see that by adding butter or margarine you can boost your calorie consumption dramatically. Try enjoying bread or toast with little or no spread. It may not taste as good, but right after you consume it, you'll be glad you did.

Many people on diets avoid drinking water

because they're afraid it will bloat them and increase their weight. This is a big mistake because your body quickly eliminates any water it doesn't need. You should drink an eight ounce glass of water at least six to eight times per day. This will increase the feeling of fullness which can help curb your appetite. In addition, the female body is 55 to 65 percent water while the male body is 65 to 75 percent water. This fluid must be replenished daily to assure good health. This is especially true for someone who's very active. Drinking water also aids the digestive process and flushes out waste products. Therefore, it is wise to drink one or two glasses of water before each meal.

Try not to eat unless it's a planned meal or snack. Learn to say no when you are offered a cookie or unwanted snack. A good line to use when offered something you don't want is, "Thank you, I'll have some in a few minutes". I heard of a lady who couldn't say no when offered something to eat. Whenever she went to a party, she would wear a loose fitting skirt or slacks with big pockets. She pinned a large sandwich bag in her pocket and after taking food, when no one was looking, she would slip the food into her pocket, and throw it in the trash when she arrived home. Some people would say this is going to extremes. However, she was committed to controlling her weight and used her creativity to compensate for her lack of ability to say no when offered food. It's not how you do it that counts, it's the result.

When you do give in and eat too much, make adjustments in your calorie intake for the rest of the day. Don't skip meals, just eat less. If you skip a meal you could become starved and may stuff yourself later.

If you eat more calories than you planned, exercise as soon as possible. For example, if you give in and eat a piece of pie the neighbor brought over, go out for a nice long walk. When you arrive home, you'll feel good since you burned off the extra calories contained in the pie.

Whenever tempted to eat an unplanned meal, try to wait 15 minutes before actually eating it. I can remember many times when someone in my office would offer me a doughnut I didn't want, insisting I take it. I would take it into my office to eat later. I would then give it to someone else or throw it away. Why should we eat something that is against our weight control program just because someone asks us to? People who are in control of their weight usually don't give into temptation very often or they wouldn't be in control of their weight. That's just a fact! The taste of food is very short lived, but, the result of eating the food can last a long time.

It is important for good health to have fiber in your diet. Some research has indicated that eating fiber with the component psyllium found in oat bran, barley, rye, fruits and vegetables may help reduce your appetite.

Be careful when you use artificial sweeteners, that you aren't playing games with yourself. Don't assume that by saving calories with artificial sweeteners; you can have that extra cookie or slice of pizza.

You may have heard frozen vegetables are less nutritious than fresh ones. The facts prove that frozen and fresh vegetables are comparable nutritionally. Vegetables are usually frozen as soon as they are brought in from the field, which seals in the nutrients. However, it can take days for fresh vegetables to get from the field to your table. Therefore, frozen vegetables are usually as nutritious, or even more nutritious than fresh ones. There is one exception and that is when fresh produce is purchased locally, in season, and eaten when they are ripe. This is the healthiest choice of all.

Avoid "FAD DIETS" which advocate eating large amounts of only one type of food (like meat, grapefruit, or nuts) for several days or weeks. You won't learn about the importance of sensible eating. When you go off the "FAD DIET" you will have the same bad eating habits and will probably gain back any weight you may have lost.

Finally, you may have heard that you should never diet when there are stressful situations in your personal life. There are studies showing that people who are under stress are actually more successful at losing weight than people whose lives are stable. This may happen because they have less time to think about eating. THE PROPER FOOD IN MODERATION WILL CURE YOUR OVEREATING PROBLEMS.

7 You Can Do Almost Anything

The date was January 21, 1986. I had received a telephone call just a few days before and had quickly made reservations to fly to San Diego, California. The only questions I had been asked was "Would my schedule permit me to be gone for three days and did I have claustrophobia?"

I arrived at the hotel in San Diego just in time to have a late dinner and go to bed. The following morning I met seven others in the hotel lobby. We were picked up in a van and taken for about a half hour drive. After we were briefed, we were met by two eight passenger twin engine aircraft. We had been issued funny looking hats which looked like a combination of ear phones and old style football helmets.

Half of us climbed aboard one aircraft and the other half boarded the other. Soon the twin engines came to life and in a few short minutes we were airborne.

Immediately we were over the Pacific Ocean. We were seated facing the rear of the aircraft with only the pilots facing forward. The seating and cabin area were quite cramped. The ocean had a beautiful blue tint to it as I looked out the round, porthole style, window beside my seat.

About an hour and a half into our flight, I noticed a wide green line in the water. It stretched out over the water as far as I could see. Our aircraft began to make quick adjustments and we started to loose altitude. My eyes were glued to the water, when suddenly the plane was just a few feet above what appeared to be pavement. The two engines went back to full power, and we hit the pavement, bounced up and were airborne again. We had missed our landing! Within seconds I observed an amazing scene. There, just outside my window, was the tower of the USS Ranger aircraft carrier. Words can not adequately express this incredible sight. I think the last time I felt this kind of awe was the first time I saw the Grand Canyon in all its majesty. We flew back around for another try. This time I was more prepared. When our wheels hit the deck with engines running at full power, we caught the cable and came to a quick stop. A very quick stop! However, we weren't jerked around much since we were seated backwards. We just sank deeper into our seats.

Within seconds we exited the aircraft and were

escorted to the bridge where we met the Captain. He presented the members of our group with a card indicating we had made an arrested landing on an aircraft carrier at sea! During the next twenty-four hours we were given tours of this city at sea. The community of 5,000 sailors on board the USS Ranger functioned the way any small town does. There were doctors, barbers, cooks, store clerks, choir directors, etc.

During our tour, I was surprised to discover that exercise was an important part of the sailors daily life. Most of the Navy personnel appeared to be in excellent shape. When we were escorted to the hanger deck, just below the flight deck where the planes are parked and maintained, I noticed groups of sailors in normal workout clothing doing calisthenics and jogging from one end of the ship to the other. There were several instructors who were leading different exercise classes. The pilots were particularly involved with exercise and weight control. They loved flying jets, and they understood that to continue flying, strict physical tests had to be passed. In other words, their goal to continue flying was so important that they were willing to work hard to stay physically fit and maintain weight control.

That night we observed what the Navy calls Night Operations. We stood on the landing deck just a few yards from where Navy F-14 Tomcat and F-18 Hornet fighter aircraft took off and landed. It was incredible how these high performance aircraft were able to land on top of the small rolling deck of the USS Ranger, even after dark. Not once did we see a fighter miss a landing. To me it seemed impossible, but the pilots, along with all of the support people, proved YOU CAN DO ALMOST ANYTHING IF YOU WANT TO BAD ENOUGH!

This is true in almost any area. If you look at people who have achieved greatness, you will almost always discover a person who has overcome failure. In fact, failure seems to be an unfair advantage. My high school swimming coach once told me a story about overcomming failure that I'll never forget.

Jeff Farrell was from Wichita, Kansas. His goal was to compete for the United States in the Olympic Games. He had been competing since he was a small boy, specializing in the 100 meter freestyle. At the 1956 Olympic Trials Jeff had failed to make the team by .1 of a second. Since competitive swimmers usually end their careers upon completion of college, and since the Summer Olympics are held every four years, the Olympic window of opportunity usually comes around only once for every swimmer. However, Jeff decided he'd try again in 1960.

To qualify for the Olympic trials, he had to have one of the best times in the country in one of the events. The trials are a very grueling and competitive experience and like the Olympics, there are no second chances. Jeff was one of the best American freestylers, and had been invited to go to the trials in Detroit. He specialized in the 100 and the 200 meter freestyle.

Jeff arrived in Detroit a week before the trials; just

three days earlier he had established new American records in the 100 and the 200 meter freestyle. This all took place at the National Outdoor AAU Championships. His plan was to continue practicing and get the general feel of the Olympic Trial pool environment. Six days before the 100 freestyle preliminaries, at about 4:15 in the morning, one of Jeff's roommates heard a crash and found Jeff on the floor of their bathroom.

Jeff's coach was summoned and Jeff was immediately rushed to the hospital. A few hours later an emergency appendectomy was performed. All hope was lost for the young swimmer since the trials were to be held in just six days, and Jeff's doctor had advised him he couldn't swim for at least three weeks. The next Olympic Games wouldn't be held for four years, and Jeff was too old to train another four years.

Two days later, Jeff, with the help of his coach, convinced his doctors to allow him to get into the hospital's pool. Over the next few days Jeff was able to slowly start swimming and overcome the severe pain. Just prior to the 100 meter freestyle preliminaries, he got approval from his doctors to try to qualify for the Olympic Team.

The Olympic Swimming Committee made a major exception and offered to allow Jeff to go to the Olympic training sight as the seventh man on the 800 meter relay team. He would later swim against the sixth man to see who would swim on the relay. This meant someone who had trained with the team would have to stay home but Jeff didn't want anyone to endure that heartache. He decided to try to make it on his own or not go at all.

On the day of the 100 meter freestyle all the swimmers reported to their starting blocks dressed in their competitive swim suits. But one swimmer was dressed a little differently. Sticking out from under his suit, was a large white bandage. Jeff swam in two preliminary races and qualified for the 100 meter finals the following day. The crowd cheered as Jeff stepped up on the starting blocks as his name was called for the 100 meter freestyle finals. The story of his appendectomy had made news all over the country. Jeff was not able to bend over in the normal starting position due to pain and the large white bandage. When the starting gun sounded, Jeff sprang off the blocks and stretched out as best he could to meet the water. His expression was one of apprehension and pain. After the turn, Jeff was in the lead, though the race was close. Then something terrible happened. Jeff's arm hit the rope. It was just enough to allow two other swimmers to finish ahead of him. One swimmer beat him by only .1 of a second. Since only the two fastest swimmers qualify for the individual events, Jeff missed qualifying and a chance for a 100 meter freestyle gold medal in Rome.

Jeff still had one more chance to make the team. If he placed sixth or better in the 200 meter freestyle the following day, he would qualify for a spot on the relay team. The 200 meter freestyle is four lengths of the pool and three painful turns. The next day Jeff qualified for the finals which consisted of the eight best qualifying times. This time things turned out differently, and as the announcement was made over the public address system that Jeff had the fourth fastest time, the crowd cheered for five minutes. Jeff's dream of making the Olympic team had come true!

Later in Rome Jeff swam the anchor leg on the 400 meter medley relay and the 800 meter freestyle relay. The United States won the gold medal, setting the American, Olympic and World record in both races.

Most people would have given up, but Jeff Farrell turned his handicap into victory. You may have been battling your weight for many years, but it's important to know you can control your weight if you want to badly enough. Feeling sorry for yourself won't work. You must want to control your weight and make it a major goal.

I remember when I was a little boy, my mother used to read a book to my sister and me before we went to bed. It was a cute little story called "The Little Engine that Could" by Watty Piper. Perhaps you are familiar with the book. It's a story about a locomotive that is pulling several railroad cars full of toys to be delivered to boys and girls in a small town. In order to deliver the toys the engine must pull the cars over a huge mountain.

The engine breaks down before it gets to the mountain and can't go any further. Some of the toys get out and try to convince another engine to pull the cars over the mountain, so the children wouldn't be disappointed the following day. After a big powerful freight train and a fast passenger engine refuse to help, the toys ask a little switch engine who has never been out of the railroad yard to help.

The little engine does not want the children to be disappointed and agrees to try to pull the cars over the mountain. The little switch engine hooks up to the cars and slowly begins to move. When they reach the mountain, the slope increases and the going gets harder and harder. The little engine says to himself over and over again, "I THINK I CAN, I THINK I CAN, I THINK I CAN, and pulls the cars very slowly over the mountain. When the train reaches the top of the mountain and starts down, the little engine says to itself over and over again, "I THOUGHT I COULD, I THOUGHT I COULD, I THOUGHT I COULD."

To successfully control your weight, it's very important to have a positive and realistic attitude. When the going gets tough don't get discouraged, learn from each challenge. Keep in mind that you can control your weight if you want to. You must THINK YOU CAN! When you are successful and reach your ideal weight, you too can proudly say, "I THOUGHT I COULD!"

Continually examine your own attitude toward weight control. Is it positive or negative? Do you think of yourself as fat or do you think of yourself as a person who controls their weight? Do you see yourself accomplishing your goals in life or do you see yourself failing? Ask yourself, if I continue to represent myself in a particular way, what will likely be the final result of my life? If the result is not what you want, change your attitude.

This whole concept is really quite simple. Lets say you have a real craving for chocolate, and every time you come in contact with chocolate you find yourself eating it. To overcome this temptation, try telling yourself you don't like chocolate. To add more power, tell other people you used to like chocolate but you really don't care for it anymore. If you maintain a positive attitude, you may soon find that resisting chocolate is no problem. In fact, many people may ask how you resist eating chocolate!

Keep in mind, that a belief is a strong emotional state of certainty that you hold about specific people, things, ideas, or experiences. However, just because you believe an idea doesn't necessarily make it true. In fact many of the beliefs you have right now are not true at all. We are all full of beliefs that are not correct. Yet our beliefs play a major role in our successes and failures.

When a great major league baseball player steps to the plate, he does not picture himself striking out. Instead, he sees himself as a great hitter who is concentrating on getting another hit. Most baseball players don't even bat .300 which means they fail more than seventy-percent of the time. Yet .300 is considered an outstanding batting average. If a player steps up to the plate thinking his chances are more than seventy-percent that he will fail, then he probably will fail almost every time. A positive attitude is necessary to accomplish most goals and objectives in life.

I remember when I was taking a speech class in high school, the first rule was not to get up in front of the audience and say, "I'm not a good speaker but..." and then go on with the speech. This is not only the wrong attitude for the speaker, but it also puts the audience in the wrong frame of mind. Instead, the speaker should step up to the podium feeling he or she has a very important message to convey to the audience and then commence to deliver that message with confidence.

The choice is up to you. You can see yourself as a person who controls your weight or a person who's weight controls you. The fact is that other people can control their weight and so can you. THE CHOICE IS YOURS!

This brings me to another point. Too often when people are looking for a cause or solution they quit after they find an answer. Many times they will defend this answer with a closed mind. However, one of the rules of creative thinking is to always look for the second, third and even the forth right answer. After examining all of the right answers, select the best one.

Probably the best way to illustrate this point is with a joke I heard sometime ago. The joke goes like this: There was a young actor who had just graduated from theatrical school. His goal was to be an actor in Hollywood. He asked his teacher what was the best way to get started. His instructor advised him to move to California and sign up at various studios.

The young actor promptly moved to Hollywood. After getting an apartment he went to several movie studios, signing up so he could be considered for a role. Many of the studios requested his clothing sizes in case they needed a person to fit a particular costume.

Sure enough, the following morning he got a call from one of the studios about a play opening that evening, and one of the bit part actors had called in sick. It was a medieval play, and the young actor's clothing size was the same as the sick actor's so the costume would fit. Upon enthusiastically accepting, he was told to report for makeup at 6:00 PM. He was then told his part would be the following: At the end of the first act, just at the right moment, he would be instructed to walk out on the stage and say "I hear the sound of the cannon." The curtain would then go down, and the first act would end. His performance would then be over.

The young actor practiced his line all day. First he practiced out loud, "I hear the SOUND of the cannon". No, that wasn't quite right. Then he tried, "I hear the sound of the CANNON." No, that wasn't right either. Then he tried, "I hear the SOUND of the CANNON!" That sounded great. So he went around his apartment all day saying out loud, "I here the SOUND of the CANNON!"

Finally, the time came for him to report to the

studio. He arrived right on schedule and reported to the director who shook hands with him and immediately asked him to recite his line. The young actor said, "I hear the SOUND of the CANNON!" The director thought he did such an outstanding job that he commented, "That was even better than the original actor. Say it exactly that way... this will be a great way to end the first act." He then took the actor to the makeup area telling him to report back to him at 7:30 PM.

After some idle conversation, the person applying the makeup asked the young actor what his line in the play was, whereupon the young actor blurted out, "I hear the SOUND of the CANNON!" "That is fantastic", replied the makeup artist. "You are going to be a great actor." After the makeup was complete the young actor slipped into his costume. It was a perfect fit. He then went around to the backstage area and practiced his line. "I hear the SOUND of the CANNON!" he said over and over again. Almost everyone who heard him offered their congratulations on his outstanding delivery.

At the prearranged time the young actor reported back to the director who asked him to stay with him throughout the first act. At just the right time the director would tell him to walk out to the center of the stage and recite his line.

The play opened and the audience responded with great appreciation. It was obvious the play was going to be a big success. Finally the young actor's performance was just one minute away and the director turned to him and said, "Lets hear your line one more time," whereby the young actor said, "I hear the SOUND of the CANNON!" The director congratulated him and said, "PERFECT!, Wait for my cue and go out on the stage and say it exactly that way, I'm going to give you the role permanently."

When the right moment arrived, the director turned to the young actor and said, "Now". The young actor walked out on the stage. Just as he arrived at center stage there was a loud BOOM! The young actor, with a startled look, jumped straight up in the air and screamed, "WHAT WAS THAT!!!!!!"

I used this joke to illustrate a very important point. The reason it's funny is that at the end of the story you discover the SECOND RIGHT ANSWER. The second right answer is what makes any joke funny. It becomes funny when you see "another" way of looking at something. As you look for the best way to control your weight, look for the second, third and forth right answers. Don't quit too soon!

8 Exercise

Exercise can be an important aid to weight control while delaying many of the declining effects that accompany aging. It can also improve your physical and mental well-being. Research has shown that you can exercise at any age with positive benefits. If you can move, you can move against resistance and stimulate your muscles to grow.

Exercise helps reduce inches off your body while making it more firm, even if your weight remains the same. Following exercise, some studies indicate that a person's metabolic rate will remain elevated for up to 12 hours, causing the body to burn even more calories throughout the day.

Commitment to exercise is one of the important

factors of weight control success. First of all, exercise speeds up your metabolic rate causing your body to burn calories more efficiently. Secondly, exercise can build muscle and tone your body. Fitness encompasses the whole body. Therefore, you should exercise a variety of body parts.

There are some important points to remember about exercise. First, you should consult your physician prior to beginning an exercise program. Secondly, stop exercising if you feel bad or become overly fatigued. Finally, if you feel like you may be coming down with a cold, cut back on your exercise routine. If you exercise too hard, you may wear down your body to the point that it will not be able to fight off a cold.

Many people think they should stretch prior to exercising. This is not correct. While stretching without bouncing is important, always warm up first. Muscles work best when their temperature is around 101 to 102 degrees Fahrenheit. Stretching cold muscles increases the risk of tearing microscopic muscle fibers which in turn damages supporting tendons and ligaments. Always warm up by walking briskly or by jogging slowly for at least five minutes. Then stretch slowly, without bouncing, for about ten minutes. Stretch all major muscle groups in your shoulders, chest, thighs, calves, and Achilles tendons. Hold each stretch for thirty seconds, but never to the point of pain. This helps maintain range of motion and flexibility. You should also stretch after you exercise when your muscles are still warm. It is important to "cool down" after exercising because this keeps your muscles from tightening while allowing a gradual return to your normal heart rate.

It is also important to drink water while you are exercising. Don't wait until you get thirsty before drinking water. If you get too thirsty your heart will be forced to work harder. This may cause you to slow down or stop early. Severe dehydration is a dangerous condition that can lead to heatstroke. Don't wait until you feel thirsty, drink water regularly during exercise.

The type of exercise you do is as important to your weight control plan as the way you exercise. To illustrate this point, let me give you a personal example. For many years I exercised five days a week, jogging six miles each day. Through the years I continued to improve my time to the point that I began running rather than jogging. At times, when I wanted to lose weight, I would either run faster or increase my distance. Following my workout, it took several minutes before my breathing went back to normal. I noticed that after running I would lose three to four pounds. I lost mostly water weight, but after five or six miles I was obviously burning calories too. The next day I would get on the scales and discover that I hadn't lost any weight. After a week, I still wasn't losing weight. I also noticed that I had a much larger appetite than normal.

I decided to try walking fast instead of running. I increased my exercise time though I actually walked a shorter distance than I normally ran. I often walked with a friend and we had a nice visit during our walk. Soon I noticed my weight going down, and I was not as hungry as I was when I ran. Why was I losing weight when I walked but not when I ran?

Here is the reason. In its simplest form, when it comes to burning calories, there are 2 types of exercise. Exercise that burns fat and exercise that burns carbohydrates. You may be aware of carbohydrate loading. This is used especially by marathon runners. The day before competition marathon runners will eat large amounts of carbohydrates such as spaghetti. They do this because, when they compete the next day, they will be exerting large amounts of energy over a long period of time. When the body is stressed, it burns the calories which are easiest to burn. These are the calories that come from carbohydrates. Therefore a workout that is too strenuous will result in burning mostly carbohydrate calories and not fat calories.

If you want to burn fat calories, exercise slowly for a longer period of time. A good rule of thumb to follow is to see if you can carry on a normal conversation, after warming up. If so, you are burning fat. On the other hand, if you can not carry on a normal conversation because you are out of breath, you are burning mostly carbohydrate calories. In weight control, we are not concerned with conditioning as much as burning fat calories. So remember, don't exercise beyond the point where you can carry on a normal conversation. This is a very important point to keep in mind while you're exercising.

You may have heard of spot weight loss. This is burning fat off a particular part of your body. It would be nice if we could spot reduce, but it just isn't possible. The only way to lose fat is to burn more calories than you eat. Your body will then naturally burn fat in its own way. You can't select the fat your body will burn first.

The building of muscle mass increases your metabolic rate. Therefore, you burn more calories as you increase the muscle mass in your body. For example, you can began an exercise program that builds your abdominal muscles. However, exercising a muscle has no direct effect on the fat around it. You will not see your strengthened muscles until you lose the fat around them. Your enlarged abdominal muscles will, however, increase the amount of calories your body burns by a small amount.

If you are trying to tone up your body, you must lose fat. To further improve tone you can build strength and muscle mass, in a particular area, through exercise or weight training. Some people are afraid to build muscle because they feel it will turn to fat once they quit. This is not true. Muscle tissue is different than fat tissue and is not capable of becoming fat tissue. If you don't exercise a muscle it will atrophy or get smaller, but it will not turn to fat. In fact, if you diet without exercising, chances are 10 to 30 percent of the weight you lose will be lean muscle tissue. Sedentary adults will lose an average of five to six pounds of muscle every 10 years even when not dieting since muscle atrophies when it is not used.

Exercise that builds muscle compensates for the muscle tissue we naturally lose as we get older. Remember, a more muscular body is more efficient in burning fat.

If at all possible, do some strength training. Calisthenics or lifting weights will build strength, increase bone density and protect against injury. Focus on muscle groups that your aerobic exercise neglects. For example, if you walk or bicycle, then concentrate on your upper body and trunk. If you have limited strength, modified calisthenics like kneeling push-ups or half sit-ups could be used. If you are fit, do exercises that pinpoint major muscle groups including the arms, shoulders, upper back, abdomen, hips and legs.

There are lots of opportunities to do calisthenics. You don't necessarily have to do them all at one time. As a young boy I enjoyed watching football games on television. While watching these games at home, rather than getting up during the commercials and getting a snack, I would do sit-ups. I would continue doing sit-ups until the commercials were over. Except during half time, I kept up this routine until the game was over. I didn't do a large number of sit-ups at one time since the commercial usually lasted about 60 seconds. However the sit-ups added up in the hundreds by the time the game was over.

When I did my homework in the evenings, I would take a break about every half hour. Rather than get something to eat, I would do calisthenics. I would alternate between sit-ups and push-ups. I did the calisthenics for two minutes then went back to my homework. Obviously my circulation picked up during the exercise and I was more alert when I continued my studies.

In my junior high school physical education classes I was soon able to do more sit-ups than anyone else in the class. My stomach was as hard as a rock. I continued this routine all the way through school.

I'll never forget the day I was doing my student teaching at a local high school. I was teaching physical education, and we were doing the testing for the President's Physical Fitness Test. We had been given a double period in order to complete the test. The students were complaining that the test was too much work. I decided to make an agreement with them so they wouldn't think they had to do all the work. If they all tried as hard as they could on the test, I would try to do 500 sit-ups after they finished and before the class bell rang.

They must have wanted to see me suffer because they began taking the President's Physical Fitness Test with renewed vigor. When they had finished I got on the mat and began doing my sit ups. I really had no idea how many I could do. Finally the bell rang and I stopped. I had completed 1,015 sit-ups.

To further illustrate the point of what happens if you continue to do a few exercises several times a day, I'll continue the sit-up story. As Co-Captain of the Washburn University swim team, I was often in the weight area of the field house doing stretching exercises prior to going to the pool. One afternoon there was a group of football players in the weight area. Most appeared to weigh well over 200 pounds. I weighed about 155 pounds. The football players were doing sit-ups holding a 25 pound weight behind their head while another football player held their ankles down. I watched as each player had a teammate lift one of the 25 pound weights into position so that he could hold it next to his head and attempt to do sit-ups. Most of the players couldn't do any, however a few did two or three sit-ups. The players yelled to encourage their teammates who were able to do at least one sit-up and booed those who failed in their attempts.

After I had watched for a few minutes, one of the players jokingly asked me if I'd like to try. I agreed and got down on the mat. He recommended I try a 10 pound weight, but I insisted on one of the 50 pound weights. After trying to discourage me, several of the players helped position the 50 pound weight behind my head. I proceeded (to their amazement) to do 10 sit-ups with the 50 pound weight. I'll never forget the look of wonder on their faces when I finished. What I didn't tell them was that I had a splitting headache from the 50 pound weight banging against my head after each sit-up. My arms were barely strong enough to hold the 50 pound weight behind my head, yet; again, by exercising on a a regular basis over a long period of time, you can develop very strong muscles!

One aspect of exercise that is often overlooked is the importance of exercising equal and opposing muscles. To illustrate this point I would again like to draw from one of my personal experiences. As I mentioned before, for many years I jogged six miles a day, Monday through Friday, on the indoor track at the local YMCA. Though I was in excellent condition, I pulled a muscle in my leg once or twice a year. This happened over and over again for a period of about 10 years, and each time I was forced to quit running until the pain went away. The reason for the pulled muscles remained a mystery.

One day during a meeting of my local civic club we had a speaker who was both a real estate executive and an athletic trainer. As a hobby he worked with top college and professional athletes during their off seasons. During his presentation he discussed how he was currently working with one major league baseball player who wanted to increase his hitting power. He pulled a muscle in his shoulder on several occasions which prevented him from hitting the ball as well as he had previously.

Our speaker told how he had the hitter swing a baseball bat backwards and simulated this same backward swing using pulley weights. The objective was to strengthen the equal and opposing muscles. He theorized that when a muscle gets too strong, and the opposing muscle is not strengthened, pulled or strained muscles will result. By the time the muscles have healed, strength will have been lost and the muscles can work together again. If the opposing muscle is not strengthened the whole process will be repeated again and again.

I decided to try this principle with my jogging. I jogged six miles as usual and then immediately jogged a forth of a mile backwards. This took some getting used to physically. In addition I had a lot of comments from other members of the YMCA. I quickly discovered that jogging backwards was much more difficult than jogging forward: it required more concentration as well as coordination. This difficulty was compounded by jogging backwards when I was tired. I switched to a new routine consisting of warming up by jogging one-fourth of a mile forward followed by jogging one-forth of a mile backward. I then did my stretching exercises followed by my six mile jog. I continue to do this routine prior to my regular workouts. Since running backwards for more than 10 years I have not pulled one muscle, and my legs have gained substantial strength.

For sometime I was kidded at the YMCA for jogging backwards. Then one Fall morning one of my friends, who had resisted the backwards theory, came up to me and said he was going to start running quarter miles backwards. When I asked him why he changed his mind, he told me he was on the campus of the University of Kansas walking down the wide, rather steep half mile hill that leads to the football stadium when he literally had to run for his life; the Jayhawk Football team was running up the hill-BACKWARDS! He later told me they were doing this to strengthen their equal and opposing muscles.

Since I began experimenting with the concept of building the equal and opposing muscles more and more people have followed suit at the YMCA because they have seen successful results. On any given day you will see people jogging and pedaling the stationary bicycle backwards. The feedback I have received has been extremely positive.

Because walking does not strain the leg muscles as much as jogging, it is not as important to walk backwards. However, it's important to keep the concept in mind should you have problems with pulled or strained muscles.

If you decide to jog backwards I want to caution you, be very careful! Jogging backwards is much more difficult, and you could fall or run into something. Be safe, not sorry!

Since exercise is so important in weight control, I'd like to illustrate another point about injuries that can effect your ability to exercise. As you exercise you are putting stress on various parts of your body in order to make them stronger. If you put added stress on a part of your body during normal daily activities, you could develop an injury. It can be difficult to discover the cause of such problems.

For example, in 1972 I developed a sore hip while jogging. It was not bad enough to keep me from working out, but it was irritating. I did everything I could to discover what was causing the soreness but to no avail. This continued until sometime in the middle of 1974. Then almost overnight, the problem went away.

The same problem surfaced again in 1983. I tried everything I could think of to correct the problem including exercising the equal and opposing muscles. I even ran laps sideways on the indoor running track at our YMCA. This is how basketball players build up their legs to improve their lateral speed. But nothing seemed to help. My hip bothered me when I walked but it was not bad enough to keep me from jogging.

In 1985 I got an idea that quickly solved my hip injury. In 1972 I had purchased a small car which was very low to the ground. I sold it in 1974 for a station wagon which I drove until 1983. In 1983, I purchased another car that was also low to the ground. Every time I got in and out of the low cars, I was putting extra pressure on my left hip. This was enough to irritate my hip, but; since it was part of my normal routine, it never occurred to me that the problem was related to my car and not to my jogging.

To solve the problem, rather than get rid of the 1983 low standing car, I turned sideways and got in and out of the car using the strength of both of my legs instead of allowing my left hip and knee to carry my weight. Within one week after changing the way I entered and exited my car my hip problem was gone.

If you develop a soreness while exercising, examine everything you do to see if there might be something which irritates the part of your body that is injured. Don't give up until you discover the reason for it. You might be very surprised when you uncover the cause of your problem.

If you do sustain an injury don't lay off, take up another activity while the injury heals. For example, if you injure a knee while running, exercising in water will maintain your muscle tone and conditioning while the knee heals. In turn, you will get back on the track quicker. You can make the comeback much easier if you don't stop exercising altogether.

There are ways to increase your exercise almost everyday. Take the stairs instead of the elevator. Get off the bus a few blocks before your destination, or have your ride let you out a few blocks early. Gradually increase the distance and speed at which you walk. Make a "walk date" instead of a lunch date. For an evening out, choose dining and dancing instead of just dinner. Ride an exercise bike while you read or watch TV. You could ride the exercise bike while talking on the telephone. (Remember, you should be able to carry on a normal conversation while burning fat calories.) Carry your own groceries from the supermarket whenever possible, this will give you a mini-muscle building workout. These fat-burning activities can add up to several additional minutes of exercise by the end of each day.

Too many people try dieting without exercise. They lose fat, but they also lose muscle. If possible it is best to combine dieting with exercise. In fact, exercise creates its own mind-set. After you go for a walk or a jog you may think, "I'm not going to blow it now by eating junk food!" Incidentally, studies of lab animals show that active animals choose a diet lower in fat than animals that don't exercise.

The psychological benefits of exercise are important to weight conscious people. Exercise decreases stress and relieves tensions which could lead to overeating. Exercise builds physical fitness, self-confidence, enhances self-image, and gives you a positive outlook on life. When you begin to feel good about yourself, you will be more likely to make positive changes in your lifestyle that will assist you with your weight control.

In addition, exercise can be fun, provides recreation, and offers opportunities for socialization. The exhilaration and emotional release received while exercising can be a boost to your mental and physical health. Pent-up anxieties and frustrations seem to disappear while you are exercising. Try to set aside a regular time to exercise and make room for it in your daily schedule. I exercise early in the morning prior to going to my office. I used to exercise immediately after work, but many times last minute telephone calls would make it impossible. Select a time that works best for you.

Be sure to choose an exercise program you will enjoy. It's easier to stick with an exercise program if you are having fun, even though it takes time and energy. There is no best exercise, so pick ones that work for you. Soon you will begin to feel better, look better, and you will experience a new enthusiasm and joy for life! You will be rewarded many times over for your efforts.

Remember, while you are exercising, think about the positive rather than the negative. If you are jogging, walking or riding a bicycle for thirty minutes, after exercising for 10 minutes, say to yourself, "I have ALREADY finished 10 minutes," or, "I ONLY have 20 minutes left." This is better than saying to yourself, "I have only exercised for 10 minutes, or, "I still have a WHOLE 2O minutes left before I'm finished." Try thinking about the positive side and notice how much better you feel!

The key is to burn fat when exercising. Do longer periods of exercise and make sure that you are able to maintain a normal conversation. This type of exercise is usually more enjoyable. To burn even more calories, carry some hand-held weights or use ankle weights while you walk. They won't make much difference in the calories you'll burn, but every little bit helps.

9 Grazing

Losing or maintaining your weight requires eating the correct amount of calories and grams of fat. However, when you eat is just as important as what you eat. The ideal weight control program requires that you don't get real hungry and develop a low blood sugar level.

To keep from being hungry or storing much of your food as fat, eat your allowed calories throughout the day. Do not skip meals or have a large meal. Make sure you eat a minimum of three meals every day. It's better to have six meals. Eating six times not only helps eliminate hunger, but also is an excellent way to enjoy food. I call this Grazing. Don't just eat six times a day, plan each snack in advance making sure to count the calories and grams of fat.

It has been found that people who eat regularly burn off ten percent more calories than people who skip meals. Every time they eat their metabolic rate goes up. By eating three or more times a day, you can burn 150 to 200 more calories than if you consumed all of your food in one meal.

Let me give you an idea of how I graze. When I get up in the morning, I have a bowl of cereal with a sliced banana on top. I select several types of dry cereal and mix them together. I always include at least one type of oat bran cereal, being sure to watch the calories and grams of fat. There is a big difference in brands. Try to stay at or below three grams of fat per serving. I discovered several years ago that if I use hot water instead of milk it tastes just as good and is much better for you. It is also more convenient and cheaper. The combined taste of the crunchy cereal, hot water and cool banana gets better each day. After breakfast, I go to the YMCA for my early morning workout prior to going to my office.

About mid-morning I have a snack. It usually consists of dry cereal or popcorn. I have lunch around noon. We fix lunch at the office. I generally have steamed vegetables and a turkey sandwich. During the middle of the afternoon I have another snack. I happen to enjoy different types of dry cereal, but any kind of low-fat snack is fine. I find I am not always hungry for the snack, but I have it anyway so I can spread my calories out over the day. I have dinner around 6:00 PM. Sometime between 8:00 PM and 9:30 PM I'll have another light snack. Since I spread my calories out over the entire day I don't get hungry. I'm careful not to exceed my allotted calories and grams of fat! The advantage of grazing is that you never feel hungry and you burn the calories as you are eating them. Your body never has time to store the excess calories as fat.

As you develop your own method of grazing don't skip meals, especially breakfast, lunch or dinner. You will enjoy life more and find that it's easier to stay on your weight control program. In fact, even if you eat too much at one meal, don't skip any regular meal. Instead have a lighter meal. This will keep you from developing low blood sugar.

When you eat, enjoy your favorite foods. There is no reason to go on a diet consisting of foods you don't like. In fact, eat a wide variety of foods, just don't exceed your calories and grams of fat per day. Be sure to include foods with a wide variety of tastes, textures and consistencies with your meal. If you hunger for sweets, eat something with a sweet taste as part of your meal so you won't be tempted to have a dessert after your meal when you are full. For example, if you crave ice cream, have a small dish of low-fat ice cream which isn't any more fattening than a large apple. If you want something sweet, remember sugar contains only four calories per gram, or about 16 calories per teaspoon. Sugar isn't a nutritional food. Sugar does not provide vitamins or minerals essential for good health. However, studies indicate most overweight people actually eat less sugar than thin people. The amount of sugar a person eats does not necessarily determine whether they will gain weight. It's fat that makes you fat. Therefore, if you eat sweets, try to avoid sweets with fat in them such as candy bars and ice cream.

Finally, try to combine carbohydrates with protein. Carbohydrates provide you with short term energy that burns rapidly while protein provides a long term source of energy that sustains you over a longer period of time. Grazing is the best way to eat, even after you reach your ideal weight.

If you are ready to seriously control your weight let's look at the FAT STATS method of weight control and see how you can turn your goal into reality.

10 The "Fat Stats" Method

There are some very important features that comprise a good long-term weight control program. There are also lots of "FAD DIETS," some of which are very expensive, bad for your health, and cause you to lose weight too rapidly. They produce results which are not permanent. The Fat Stats weight control method incorporates the latest weight control information and eliminates the negatives of "FAD DIETS."

Everyone is different, so never compare yourself with anyone else. Therefore, a good weight control program should be individualized just for you. You need to know your percentage of body fat. You can then determine whether you need to lose, gain or maintain your current weight. Body fat is the percentage of total body weight that is fat. For example: A male who weighs 200 pounds with 20% body fat, carries 40 pounds of fat on his body! There is no such thing as the perfect body fat percentage that applies to everyone. However, a good lifetime body fat percentage to pursue is 16% for men and 19% for women.

When a girl reaches her full growth, somewhere around age 13 to 17, and her weight is average, her body fat will be about 19%. When a boy reaches his full growth, somewhere around age 15 to 18, and his weight is average, his body fat will be about 16%. From this time on there is no need for men or women to add any additional body fat. Ideally, this percentage of body fat should be maintained throughout life.

As we get older, the average person tends to get less exercise, burn fewer calories, eat more fattening foods and therefore accumulates unneeded body fat. Therefore the average percent body fat for men and women increases as they get older. Or stated another way, if women maintain their 19% body fat as they get older, they will be leaner than average for their age group. This will continue as their age increases. A woman's ideal body fat is still 19%. The same is true for men. They should maintain 16% body fat throughout their lifetime.

When women are in their twenties, estrogen causes them to store fat in their hips and thighs. As women reach their thirties and forties, estrogen levels decline slightly. After menopause their levels of adrenal steroids increase. Since adrenals favor abdominal fat distribution, or the "apple" shape, older women may start depositing fat around their stomachs. Men always tend to store their body fat around their stomachs. As men and women store more and more fat, it begins to spread over their entire body. Remember, there is no need for men to have more than 16% body fat or women to have more than 19%. A key part of the FAT STATS weight control program is to provide each person with his individualized percent body fat.

A good weight control program should also provide you with your target weight. It is important that this is your ideal weight and not a weight that sounds good to you. It should be your exact weight to the nearest pound, rather than a weight range. It should be based on factual information-not guess work. Some popular weight control programs ask their customers what they want to weigh. This often is an inaccurate target weight.

A long term weight control program requires the knowledge of your ideal weight. This will depend on your age, sex, height, and bone structure. With FAT STATS your actual body measurements are used to determine your target weight. For women, age, height, weight, neck, forearm, wrist and hip measurements are used. For men, age, height, weight, neck and abdomen measurements are used. This is the method developed by the United States Army to determine the percent of body fat for its personel.

Since excessive body fat is a basis for discharge, it was very important for the Army to have an accurate and consistent method of figuring body fat. The Army used to use the skinfold caliper method of measuring body fat but found, even with well trained personnel, it was inconsistent. The circumference measurement method was developed to meet this need. One benefit of the circumference measurement method is that untrained people can take the measurements quite easily in the privacy of their own home. The FAT STATS program takes advantage of this new method of figuring body fat.

If you need to lose a great deal of weight, its beneficial to have your FAT STATS program redone after each 25 pounds you lose. Your measurements will have changed and your body will probably be burning fewer calories. Also people store large amounts of excess fat in slightly different ways. This will have an affect on figuring your ideal weight. As your weight approaches a more normal level, your ideal weight can be determined more accurately. It resembles the process a sculptor uses when chipping a figure out of stone. Your recheck may indicate a slightly lower ideal weight. This should not be a source of discouragement but one of encouragement as you go through the process of reaching your ideal weight and maintaining this weight throughout your lifetime.

To be successful in controlling your weight, you need to know how many calories you burn each day.

Without this information you can only guess at how many calories you should eat. The FAT STATS program will provide you with your approximate Basal Metabolic Rate (a measure of the average rate of calories burned per day if your body was in a constant resting state) and the approximate calories you burn each day based on your activity level.

It is also important to monitor the grams of fat you consume each day. Fat, besides promoting obesity, has been linked to an increased risk of developing cancer, heart disease, hypertension and diabetes. Eating fat is the quickest way to get fat. Fats in your diet appear to be converted to body fat more easily than proteins and carbohydrates. The reason is that during digestion, the body burns many more calories metabolizing protein and carbohydrates than it does metabolizing fat. For very 100 calories of carbohydrates we consume in excess of our daily requirement, only 75 are turned into body fat. However 97 of every 100 excess fat calories are turned into body fat. Most health organizations recommend that the grams of fat you consume each day should be no more than 30% of the calories you eat. Some experts are suggesting less. However, unless your physician recommends less, 30% should be adequate.

A good weight control program should also show you how to lose one pound per week. Gradual weight loss is important! You should not try to lose weight too quickly. If you start losing weight too rapidly, your body will go into metabolic shock. Metabolic shock occurs when your body thinks it is starving and slows down all of your bodily functions. This causes your body to burn fewer calories and therefore makes it harder to lose weight. It is almost impossible to lose more that three or four pounds of fat each week. Any more weight loss is water and or muscle tissue. Studies have also revealed that rapid weight loss is usually followed by rapid weight gain. By losing one pound per week, you build the feeling of success which will help build your self-confidence. Fat Stats provides you with altered daily calories and grams of fat, so you'll lose one pound per week.

In addition FAT STATS will provide you with the calories you burn per hour while walking at 3.5 miles per hour, while bicycling at 9.5 miles per hour, while doing aerobic dancing at a medium level, while swimming a slow crawl, while jogging at a 11.5 minute mile pace and while running at an 8 minute mile pace. This is based on your individual weight and metabolism. You will have the actual information you need to determine the number of calories you burn during exercise. This can help you in controlling your weight. For example, if you want to eat a piece of pie containing 350 calories, you can refer to your FAT STATS report and figure how many minutes you will need to exercise to burn the calories in the pie. When doing one of the exercises, be sure to only count the time you are actually exercising. If you are out for a walk and stop to visit with a friend, don't count the time you are visiting as exercise time.

Finally, a good weight control program should give you a customized body fat ratings chart so you can see how you compare with other people your same age and sex. You will then be able to follow your progress as your weight changes. The FAT STATS report gives you a detailed, individualized BODY FAT RATINGS CHART.

With the FAT STATS weight control method, you have all the critical information needed to effectively control your weight. My FAT STATS Personalized Body Profile is illustrated on page 116.

11 Food Labels

Listing the nutritional content of packaged foods is very helpful to people who are controlling their weight as well as people who are required to eat special diets by their physicians. At the time this book was printed, the federal government decided to require food labels on 270,000 items by May 1994. These labels will carry uniform information on calorie, fat, cholesterol, salt, carbohydrate and protein content. They will restrict the use of terms such as "light in fat" to denote a product's fat content or "light in salt" to denote a product's salt content. Terms such as light can mean literally anything. For example, a "light" cake might simply refer to having a lighter texture.

This information will allow consumers to

compare nutrients in a food product with their dietary needs. This is based on a daily diet of 2,000 calories and 65 grams of fat. As companies are required to provide this information they will be forced by competition to make their products more nutritious.

Though the government has not released the exact requirements the labels should contain the following information:

Nutrition Facts

Serving Size 1/2 cup (114g)
Servings Per Container 4

Amount Per Serving	
Calories 260	Calories from Fat 120
	% Daily Value*
Total Fat 13g	**20%**
Saturated Fat 5g	**25%**
Cholesterol 30mg	**10%**
Sodium 660mg	**28%**
Total Carbohydrate 31g	**11%**
Sugars 5g	
Dietary Fiber 0g	**0%**
Protein 5g	

Vitamin A 4% • Vitamin C 2% • Calcium 15% • Iron 4%

*Percents (%) of a Daily Value are based on a 2,000 calorie diet. Your Daily Values may vary higher or lower depending on your calorie needs:

Nutrient		**2,000 Calories**	**2,500 Calories**
Total Fat	Less than	65g	80g
Sat Fat	Less than	20g	25g
Cholesterol	Less than	300mg	300mg
Sodium	Less than	2,400mg	2,400mg
Total Carbohydrate		300g	375g
Fiber		25g	30g

1g Fat = 9 calories
1g Carbohydrate = 4 calories
1g Protein = 4 calories

Don't be misled by vegetable oils labeled "no cholesterol." There is no cholesterol in any vegetable oil. However, vegetable oils such as palm or coconut can be highly saturated, and saturated vegetable oil, like animal fat, raises cholesterol levels.

The Surgeon General's report recommends we should limit our consumption of both saturated and unsaturated fats. These fats have a different chemical distinction in the make up of each fat molecule by having different numbers of hydrogen atoms. If fat contains as many hydrogen atoms as it can hold, it is considered saturated (with hydrogen). If the fat can hold additional hydrogen it is called unsaturated. Unsaturated fats are divided into monounsaturated and polyunsaturated.

Fats can be made more solid by adding hydrogen. This process is called hydrogenation. An example of this is stick margarine and soft margarine. Usually the more hydrogen added to fat or oil, the more saturated and firm it becomes.

We know that foods high in saturated fat raise cholesterol levels and contribute to heart disease. All saturated fat raises cholesterol. A rule to remember is that saturated fats are generally solid at room temperature while unsaturated fats are usually liquid at room temperature. Polyunsaturated fats are liquid at room temperature and remain liquid even when cold. Monounsaturated fats are liquid at room temperature but may become solid when cold. Olive oil is probably the best example of a monounsaturated fat since it remains clear and liquid when stored at room temperature, but it becomes cloudy and begins to solidify when stored in the refrigerator.

Saturated fats are primarily found in foods originating from animals. Dairy products including milk, cream, ice cream, sour cream, butter, cheese, lard, chicken fat and beef fat are examples of saturated fat. Saturated fats are also found in tropical oils such as coconut oil, palm oil, palm kernel oil, cocoa butter, and any other vegetable oil that has been hydrogenated.

You should be aware that saturated fats are sometimes found in processed foods such as cooking oil, salad dressing, popcorn, bakery items, bouillon cubes and some non-dairy creamers. Be a good detective and read the product label on each item.

Choose margarines that list liquid oil as the first ingredient. These are less saturated and thus are less likely to affect blood cholesterol levels.

Studies indicate that saturated fats contribute to cardiovascular disease such as heart attacks and stroke. However, high-fat diets of both saturated and unsaturated fats have been linked to cancer. In fact, research indicates that unsaturated fats seem to increase cancer risk more than saturated fats.

Since high-fat diets of both saturated and unsaturated fat have been linked to disease, the Surgeon General, heart experts, and cancer experts recommend reducing the amount of all fats in the diet.

Reading food labels carefully will help in your weight control efforts.

12 Goals

In the previous chapters, we have covered the basic knowledge needed to control your weight throughout your lifetime. However, this knowledge is not enough. It is extremely important to set goals. In fact, if we don't have goals to pursue, we quickly get bored or depressed.

I received my degree in physical education but decided to enter the life insurance business. One of the biggest problems a life insurance agent has is staying motivated. My goal was to make the Million Dollar Round Table. However, this goal always eluded me. Then one year I made a few big sales and qualified as a Provisional Applicant. To be a Qualifying member of the Million Dollar Round

Table you must qualify two years in a row.

By the middle of the next year I reviewed my production and discovered I wasn't even close to being on schedule. If I didn't qualify this year I would have to start all over. I decided I needed to develop a definite plan. One of the most important parts of the life insurance business is to see the people. In order to see the people you must schedule appointments, so I decided to schedule ten appointments per week.

If I followed this plan I would schedule about forty appointments per month which should easily allow me to qualify for the Million Dollar Round Table. I decided that if I accomplished this scheduling goal for eight weeks I would reward both myself and my family. I explained my plan to my wife and three children at the dinner table and told them we would all decide on the reward together. My family all thought this was a great idea and selected a CB Radio as our first reward.

The following day when we sat down to dinner my middle child, Shane, said "Dad - did you make your two appointments today? My handle is going to be ROADRUNNER." Fortunately, I had made the two appointments. From that time on I decided I couldn't let my family down and scheduled the ten appointments each week. Suddenly my whole family got excited about my work. Eight weeks later we went out and purchased our CB Radio. We immediately selected our next eight week reward. Each member of the family took turns choosing our reward as I accomplished each eight week goal.

To make a long story short, I continued my plan and by the end of the year I easily made the Million Dollar Round Table. I continued this concept the following year and with my success I was soon asked to speak at meetings and conventions all over the country. What I had done was break down a major goal into small parts and accomplish the goal one step at a time. My family helped me succeed and we all enjoyed the accomplishments and rewards together. Weight loss can be accomplished in the same way. Set intermediate goals, such as every five pounds, then reward yourself with a non-food reward.

Your mind is not capable of helping you succeed unless you give it a goal. The pursuit of the goal will give you the mental gratification to continue! It must be a specific goal and one with an outcome you really want. If you want to lose weight, your ultimate goal should be to attain your ideal weight. There is no reason to stop short. Don't be satisfied until you reach your goal. A FAT STATS report is the best way to find out your ideal weight.

You can reach your ideal weight! It isn't just a dream it can be a reality. Get excited about reaching your goal. See in your mind's eye how you will look when you reach your ideal weight. Step into the future and picture all the new clothes you can wear. See the changes in your stomach, face, arms and hips. Imagine how you will feel when you climb a flight of stairs. Feel the new bounce in your step as you walk down the street with your new body. Remember, experiencing an outcome is the first step in making it happen. When you realize goals in your mind, you program them into your nervous system and make them a reality.

Write down why you want to lose the weight. Give yourself reasons that are important to you. This will give your mind more ammunition as it starts guiding you towards your goal. Your mind will react to reasons why you want to lose weight even more than the techniques of shedding the extra pounds. Give yourself enough reasons, and your brain will find a way to achieve the results you want.

Always state your goals in a precise and positive way. Remind yourself that YOU are controlling your weight. Don't allow yourself to dwell on negative thoughts. One of the best ways to overcome negative thoughts is to sit or stand with good posture. I have a good friend in his seventies who continually has a very positive outlook. He always sits and stands erect with ideal posture. He has something positive to say about every situation or discussion. His positive attitude influences everyone he meets. The next time you feel discouraged, examine your posture. Sit or stand as straight as possible. Hold your head up and smile. You will be amazed at how this will change your entire outlook. Most successful people look on the positive side of any situation no matter how grim things may appear. It will help to imagine how it feels to be positive and happy. Try it, it works!

Use visualization and act as if you are already

losing weight. Be aware of the positive feelings as you tell people you are beginning a program to control your weight. Soon you and everyone will be convinced.

During the 1964 Presidential Campaign, the Democratic candidates were Lyndon Johnson and Hubert Humphrey. The Republican candidates were Barry Goldwater and William Miller. The Republican candidate for Vice President, Bill Miller, was coming to Topeka for a speech. My wife Kathy and I were interested in politics and enjoyed seeing candidates whenever they came to our city. It was a rainy morning prior to Bill's arrival, scheduled for 11:30 AM. Kathy and I parked our car at the airport at 11:00 AM. About that time the rain stopped. I decided to get out to see when the plane would arrive. Kathy, who was seven months pregnant with our first child, decided to wait in the car. I had on a business suit and a trench coat due to the inclement weather.

I walked out onto the tarmac and was immediately approached by someone who appeared to be either a secret service agent or an agent of the Kansas Bureau of Investigation. He told me only authorized personnel were allowed on the tarmac. Without thinking I replied, "I'll let you know if I see anyone that shouldn't be here." I then asked the agent when Bill's plane would arrive. He indicated he would arrive in the next few minutes and walked away. I went back to the car and informed Kathy. She got out and waited behind the fence while I went back out on the tarmac. Soon, the agent came over and informed me that Bill's plane had just landed. I noticed that the Governor's black limousine had just arrived. It was going to be used to transport Bill Miller to the sight of his speech. The security was very tight as the crowd was parted to allow the limousine to get onto the tarmac.

I heard the roar of the plane's engines and saw it make the turn onto the tarmac. To my surprise, the plane came to a stop in front of me, and the ladder came out of the plane almost hitting my foot. I noticed that I was standing between the ladder and Chet Mize, the Republican candidate for Congress. Before I could move, Bill Miller stepped out and waved to the crowd. He started walking down the ladder with his wife (Stephanie). He looked me straight in the eye and said, "Hi, I'm Bill Miller" and shook my hand. I replied, "Hi Bill, I'm Dave Fisher." Bill replied, "Dave, I'd like you to meet my wife Stephanie." I shook hands with Stephanie and said, "Bill and Stephanie, I'd like to introduce you to our Republican canditate for Congress, Chet Mize." With me in the middle, Chet Mize and Bill Miller shook hands. I looked up and noticed the press corps were rapidly taking pictures of their handshake. The Millers and Chet Mize were quickly escorted to the waiting limousine and the motorcade began to form.

I went back to join Kathy and we got into our car. I was late for an appointment and started driving through the crowd. Much to my surprise, the forming motorcade was pulling out. Leading were two highway patrolmen on motorcycles. They were followed by the Governor's limousine. The limousine was followed by a car containing security personnel. There was a short opening in the forming motorcade, and I pulled out and joined the caravan. An additional two highway patrolmen pulled in behind me on motorcycles. We picked up speed and drove through Topeka at speeds approaching 50 mph. The normal speed limit was between 20 and 35 mph. The police had blocked off each intersection along our route. Kathy looked behind and noticed the two highway patrolmen on their motorcycles followed by two large buses carrying the press corps. A police car made up the final car in the motorcade. As we drove through the streets of Topeka, crowds gathered and waved at Bill Miller as he passed. At the intersection near the hotel where Bill was to speak, the motorcade made a left turn while Kathy and I proceeded straight. I'll never forget the looks on the faces of the two highway patrolmen when they turned left while we went straight.

The following morning, I got the paper to see if my picture was on the front page with Chet Mize and Bill Miller, shaking hands while I stood between them. It wasn't there. I'm sure someone probably wondered who that person in the middle was and decided not to print the picture!

The point of this story is that if you act like you know what you are doing, you will convince everyone else including yourself. The same is true in weight control. Act like you are controlling your weight. Do the same things people do who control their weight.

Soon you will be effectively controlling your weight.

The journey in losing weight can be exciting and you should feel proud as you progress towards your ultimate goal. Feel good because you are controlling your weight. If you will commit to the ideas presented in this book, you will soon enjoy the benefits of maintaining your ideal weight for a lifetime. Remember, WHAT YOU DO TODAY WILL DETERMINE YOUR WEIGHT TOMORROW!

13 Nine Keys To Weight Control

1. Exercise is beneficial while dieting. Consult your physician before starting any diet or exercise program. The type of exercise is up to you. Remember, be able to carry on a normal conversation while exercising so you burn fat calories instead of carbohydrate calories. If you are an athlete who is trying to lose weight, be sure to do exercises that burn fat.

2. It is very important to know your personal target weight. Always keep it in mind! It is difficult to reach a goal unless you know exactly where you are and exactly where you want to be. Your target weight should be an exact weight such as 116 pounds or 158 pounds, not a range like 115-120.

3. Monitor your weight each day at the same time on the same scales. It is important to have accurate and consistent scales. It is best to have scales that will weigh you to the nearest half pound. Don't be afraid of the scales or get discouraged if your weight increases. Learn to understand why your weight changes. The scales are your feedback, they help you control your weight. You may soon know why your weight is up or down. For example, you may eat something that causes you to retain water and thus weigh more the next day even though you didn't exceed your calorie and grams of fat limit. However, after you lose the water, your weight will come down. Most women will retain water naturally at certain times each month. It's important to understand this, so you don't get discouraged when your weight is up. Just remember, it will also go down naturally. Keep a daily record so you can monitor your progress. Save your records and compare the results from year to year. You will be able to see the times of year when you have the most difficulty maintaining your weight.

4. Follow your calorie and grams of fat allowance per day to lose one pound each week. If you eat too many calories, do some activity that will burn off the extra calories. As an example, if you eat a piece of pie that puts you over your calorie limit, go for a walk that will burn the calories contained in the pie. When you finish the walk you will have a good feeling knowing you burned up the extra calories. As you monitor your weight on a daily basis, you may no longer need to count calories as you may be able to

predict your weight based on your daily exercise and food consumption.

5. Use the grazing method of eating. Eat a minimum of three well-balanced meals daily. If you get hungry before bedtime, eat fewer calories throughout the day and have a light, low-fat snack before going to bed. Some people eat up to six times a day without exceeding their calorie limit. The more times you eat the better! However, plan your meals and snacks in advance.

6. Picture how you will look and feel when you reach your target weight. Visualize yourself handling problem eating situations successfully.

7. Enjoy your favorite foods, just eat a little less and stay within your calorie and grams of fat limit per day. If you keep from eating your favorite foods you may feel deprived. This may ultimately cause you to eat larger amounts than you would have normally eaten. Take 20 minutes to eat each meal and drink plenty of water. Eat in a relaxed atmosphere.

8. Lose only one pound per week. This should be easy if you commit to your calories and grams of fat allowed per day and will help you maintain your weight once you reach your target weight. Don't try to lose weight too fast, and don't skip meals.

9. Limit alcohol intake. Alcohol contains empty calories and published research indicates it may cause bodies to burn fats more slowly. If you are going to drink alcohol, do not eat foods high in fat at the same

setting. Alcohol can cause hypoglycemia (low blood sugar) which decreases liver glucose output. Alcohol stimulates the appetite and can lower inhibitions and the ability to resist fattening foods. Ounce for ounce, alcohol has almost twice as many calories as sugar. If you also consider the calories in the mixers, you may decide your calories are better spent on more nutritious foods.

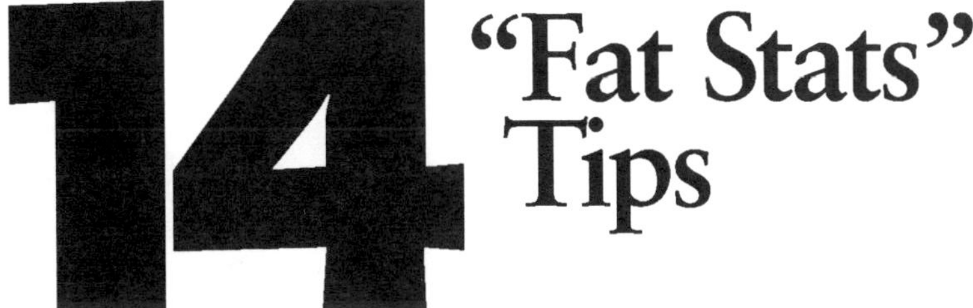

14 "Fat Stats" Tips

1. Consult your physician prior to dieting or exercising.
2. Don't start a diet that contains health risks.
3. Don't lose weight too fast. One pound per week is ideal.
4. Don't skip meals.
5. Count your calories and don't exceed your allowed calories per day.
6. Count your grams of fat and don't exceed your allowed grams of fat per day.
7. Keep a record of the calories and grams of fat you eat and when you consumed them for at least one week. This gives you valuable information regarding your eating habits. Repeat

this record keeping if you stop losing weight.

8. Keep a record of your weight each day so you can see where you were one week, one month, and one year ago.
9. Set goals in five pound increments. As you successfully reach each goal, give yourself a non-food reward.
10. Remind yourself of your goals daily.
11. Drink an eight-ounce glass of water before each meal.
12. Drink six to eight, eight-ounce glasses of water each day.
13. Add action activities to your day.
14. Exercise regularly.
15. Take the stairs whenever possible.
16. Eat oat bran. It adds bulk to the stomach's contents making you feel full, and it may help reduce serum cholesterol.
17. Eat wheat bran. It's outer covering is more than forty percent fiber, mostly insoluble which adds bulk to the contents of the intestines, this helps prevent constipation and may ward off colon cancer.
18. Watch granola-style cereals which are often high in fat because nuts and oils have been added. Many also add palm or coconut oils which are highly saturated.
19. Use brown rice instead of polished refined white rice or instant rice because it has much more fiber.
20. Stay away from frying foods. Instead broil, bake, boil, steam, grill, micro-cook, roast or

poach. Don't use sauces that contain lots of fat.

21. Eat lots of fiber and complex carbohydrates like salads and vegetables.
22. Limit adding fat-laden salad dressing. Read the labels. Vinegar or citrus juices mixed with a little seasoning makes a tangy fat-free dressing.
23. Don't cook vegetables, pasta and rice with added fat.
24. Add flavor with herbs, spices, onion, garlic, ginger or citrus juices instead of fats and salt.
25. Limit your consumption of animal protein.
26. Cut off all visible fat from meat and poultry.
27. Remove skin from poultry before or after cooking. Most of the fat lies just under the skin. Light meat has less fat than dark meat.
28. Choose lean cuts of meat.
29. When purchasing ground beef, choose the leanest available. This is often listed as ninety-five percent lean.
30. Drain off the fat after cooking beef. By using a strainer, rinse off the excess fat juices. Then add seasoning. At least blot the beef off with a paper towel.
31. Think of meat as a side dish not the main course and slice it thinly to make a serving appear more generous.
32. On hamburgers use lettuce and tomato toppings instead of mayonnaise.
33. Cook soups, stews and sauces ahead and then chill. Remove the fat after it hardens on top. Preparing dishes a day ahead also improves the

flavor.

34. Choose leaner kinds of fish like cod, flounder, haddock, halibut, orange roughy, red snapper and sole.
35. Use cocktail sauce with fish instead of tartar sauce. Cocktail sauce is a low-fat mixture of ketchup, lemon juice and horseradish. Tartar sauce is mayonnaise with chopped pickles. One tablespoon of tartar sauce has about seventy calories, and almost all of them come from fat. Imitation mayonnaise is now available with less fat and calories.
36. Steam vegetables, and use herbs and spices rather than butter or margarine.
37. When eating out at restaurants ask how foods are prepared before ordering. If sauce is included ask the waiter to leave it off or put it on the side.
38. Include lots of fruit and vegetables in your allowed calories.
39. Have low-fat snacks such as air-popped pop-corn, low-fat bran cereals, non-fat yogurt or non-fat crackers.
40. Consider having one or two vegetarian days each week.
41. Read food labels and choose the lowest fat product.
42. Buy a food scale and use it to make certain you're keeping within your allowed calories and grams of fat.
43. Watch portion sizes, they can fool you.
44. Put the food you want to eat on your plate and

don't go back for seconds. Leave the rest in the kitchen so you won't be tempted.

45. Start your meal off with a low-calorie appetizer such as a low-calorie soup, raw vegetable or fresh fruit. You will become satisfied faster and you will eat less overall.
46. EAT SLOWLY and enjoy each bite.
47. Select foods that require lots of chewing.
48. When you eat pizza, choose vegetarian pizza without extra cheese. Remember, there is no rule that you have to eat until the pizza is gone. Freeze leftovers for another meal.
49. Stay away from batter-dipped chicken or fish.
50. Potatoes are low-fat, fiber-rich foods.
51. Choose low-fat dairy products whenever possible.
52. When you stir-fry, use non stick vegetable spray.
53. Eliminate temptations by removing all high-fat foods from your refrigerator and cupboards.
54. Stock up on low-fat cereals, low-fat dairy products, fresh fruits and vegetables, and nutritious snacks that are low in fat and calories.
55. Switch from high-fat cake to angel-food cake.
56. Switch from doughnuts to bagels.
57. Read the labels on packaged vegetables carefully, as many are loaded with salt.
58. Eat fruit which is high in fiber instead of drinking fruit juice.
59. Cut up raw vegetables and fruit. Soak vegetables in ice water and sliced apples and pears in a water and lemon juice solution, to prevent them from browning.
60. Darker vegetables are usually more nutritious.

For example, large bright-orange carrots contain more vitamins than small pale carrots.

61. Avoid buying pre-cut fresh vegetables because they lose vitamins and minerals when left sitting around.
62. The longer vegetables are kept the more nutrients they lose.
63. Avoid frozen vegetables with added cream or cheese sauces, since they're high in fat and calories.
64. Limit alcohol intake.
65. Don't give up if you aren't losing weight, instead become a detective, discover why and make changes.
66. The following are 11 nutritious snacks that contain almost no calories:
    1. Raw broccoli
    2. Raw cauliflower
    3. Celery
    4. Cucumber slices
    5. Dill pickles
    6. Green peppers
    7. Lettuce
    8. Mushroom slices
    9. Radishes
    10. Soda water
    11. Zucchini

15 Conclusion

I've tried to convey throughout this book that regardless of how much you weigh now, you can enjoy the physical and psychological benefits of maintaining your ideal weight throughout your lifetime. But before you can reach your ideal weight, you must make a personal commitment. Once you make this decision you should take immediate and continuous action. Don't put it off! If you have not made a commitment to take control of your weight and change your eating habits, do it now!

After committing to take control of your eating habits, you should determine your ideal weight. The best method to accomplish this is through a FAT STATS Personalized Body Profile. The profile will not only provide you with your ideal weight, but with how many calories and grams of fat you should consume per day to lose one pound each week. It is personalized just for you. Don't skip this important step. Your mind needs a goal to achieve, and it should be as accurate as possible. An educated guess just isn't good enough. It could be way off.

Don't try to lose weight too fast. If you do, your body will think it's starving and go into metabolic shock. Your metabolism will slow down and you will have to reduce you calorie consumption even more to lose weight. The result will be increased hunger and a loss of energy. If you lose one pound per week you'll feel good and your body will not resist losing the weight.

Your weight scales are your best feedback. Weigh yourself everyday in the morning. Some people find it helpful to weigh themselves each morning and again at night. DON'T EVER GET DISCOURAGED IF YOUR WEIGHT GOES UP, LEARN WHY! Before you get on the scales, it's beneficial to your learning process, to try and predict how much you'll weigh. Before making your prediction, review in your mind everything that you did that would affect your weight since you last weighed yourself. Then, step on the scales. If your weight was higher or lower than you expected, ask yourself WHY? Soon your predictions will be correct most of the time. It's important to weigh yourself every day you possibly can, even if you know your weight will be up. Don't just weigh yourself when you think your weight is down. This is an important part of understanding how to control your weight.

Exercise is helpful in losing weight. It burns calories as well as builds or maintains muscle mass. Muscle mass is part of your lean body weight. If you don't exercise as you lose fat, you will lose some muscle mass. Since you are losing lean body weight along with fat, when you get down to your ideal weight, you will find you need to lose a little more to get your percent body fat down to 19% for women or 16% for men.

Keep using the ideas contained in this book and never go back to your old eating patterns. Pay particular attention to the information in the chapters titled CHARACTER and VISUALIZATION. Use the grazing method of eating. Eat a minimum of three times a day. It's even better for you to eat five or six times each day. Try to spread your allowed calories and grams of fat throughout your entire day.

As you have small setbacks, don't get discouraged or go on eating binges. Instead, immediately ask yourself WHY and you'll learn from your mistakes. Follow your weight control plan each day like a science and then put it out of your mind. Get plenty of exercise and get involved with life. Keep busy with your work, and do the things you enjoy doing.

Always keep in mind, WHAT YOU DO TODAY WILL DETERMINE YOUR WEIGHT TOMORROW!

Use the FAT STATS Weight Control Program, IT WORKS!

A Appendix

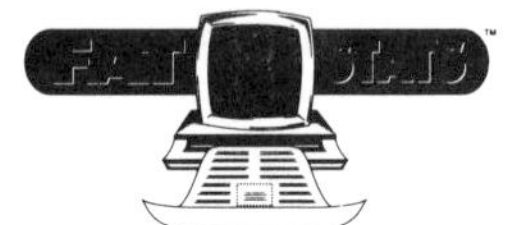

3127 SW Huntoon, Suites 1-4, Topeka, KS 66604-1600 • (913) 233-9203

```
DAVE FISHER                        AGE 52
Male                           05-18-1993
-----------------------------------------
Height    69.75     Weight     154.00
Neck      14.75     Abdomen     32.75
-----------------------------------------
YOUR PERSONALIZED BODY PROFILE
Body Fat 16%  (Very lean)
Basal Metabolic Rate              1428
Activity Level                Moderate
Calories you burn per day         1856
g of Fat per day                    62
-----------------------------------------
TO LOSE ONE POUND PER WEEK
Save/burn 500 Calories per day
Calories allowed per day          1356
g of Fat allowed per day            45
-----------------------------------------
CALORIES YOU BURN PER HOUR
Walking-3.5 mph                    333
Bicycling-9.5 mph                  416
Aerobic Dancing-moderate           425
Swimming-slow crawl                536
Jogging-11.5 minute/mile           564
Running-8 minute/mile              878
-----------------------------------------
BODY FAT RATINGS    %FAT*    WEIGHT
Very lean           12-17    147-155
Lean                18-20    157-161
Leaner than avg     21-23    163-168
Average             24-25    170-172
Fatter than avg     26-28    174-179
Fat                 29-31    182-187
Over fat            32+      190+
*Based on current measurements

  (C) Fisher Productions, Inc.
```

A good lifetime body fat target to pursue is 16% for men and 19% for women.

AT 16% YOUR TARGET WEIGHT IS: 154

1202

DAVE FISHER
3230 MACVICAR
TOPEKA, KS 66611

Definitions

YOUR PERSONALIZED BODY PROFILE

- **Body Fat %** The percentage of your total body weight that is fat. For example: A male who weighs 200 pounds, with 20% body fat, carries 40 pounds of fat on his body!
- **Basal Metabolic Rate** A measure of the average rate of calories burned per day if your body was in a constant resting state. Your Basal Metabolic Rate is based on your height and weight. Therefore the average 6'4", 200 lb. man requires more calories than the average 5'4", 110 lb. woman.
- **Activity Level**
  Active - Active lifestyle, vigorous exercise 3-5 x per wk.
  Moderate - Moderate lifestyle, exercise 3-5 x per wk.
  Light - Moderate lifestyle, light exercise
  Sedentary - Sedentary, inactive lifestyle, no exercise
- **Calories You Burn Per Day** Calories you burn per day is based on your Basal Metabolic Rate and your activity level. Besides exercise, your occupation has an effect on calories burned per day. Example: A construction worker who does little additional exercise would have an activity level comparable to an accountant who exercises 3-5 times per week.
- **g of Fat Per Day** This is 30% of calories you burn per day based on your current activity level. **(Many national health organizations recommend lowering fat intake to no more than 30% of calories.)**

TO LOSE ONE POUND PER WEEK

- **Calories Allowed Per Day** Maximum calories you may consume per day, in order to lose one pound per week, based on your current activity level.
- **g of Fat Allowed Per Day **** This is 30% of calories allowed per day.
- **Save/Burn 500 Calories Per Day** Amount of calories to be saved and or burned per day in order to lose one pound per week. This can be achieved by increasing your activity level and/or consuming fewer calories.

CALORIES YOU BURN PER HOUR

A measure of the calories you burn per hour specific to your individual body.

BODY FAT RATINGS

Body fat ratings are based on your current measurements and are specific to your individual body. **Changes that occur in your measurements will result in a new set of ratings.**

SUGGESTIONS FOR LOSING ONE POUND PER WEEK

For best results, it is recommended that you lose no more than 1 pound per week. We recommend that you consult your physician before starting any diet or exercise program.

Set realistic goals! If you want to lose 20 pounds, set goals in 5 pound increments until you meet your target weight. **(A new FAT STATS report every couple of months will help you monitor your progress as your measurements change!)**

To order a FAT STATS Personalized Body Profile, for a one time fee of $12.00 including tax and postage, call 1-800-444-7215.

FAT STATS
A division of Fisher Productions, Inc.
P.O. Box 4004
Topeka KS 66604

Price Subject to change without notice.

To order a FAT STATS Personalized Body Profile, for a one time fee of $12.00 including tax and postage, call 1-800-444-7215.